CU00794059

Dependence and Autonomy in Old Age

Respecting the autonomy of disabled people is an important ethical issue for providers of long-term care. In this influential book, George Agich abandons comfortable abstractions to reveal the concrete threats to personal autonomy in this setting, where ethical conflict, dilemma, and tragedy are inescapable. He argues that liberal accounts of autonomy and individual rights are insufficient, and offers an account of autonomy that matches the realities of long-term care. The book therefore offers a framework for caregivers to develop an ethic of long-term care within the complex environment in which many dependent and aged people find themselves.

Previously published as *Autonomy and Long-term Care*, this revised edition, in paperback for the first time, takes account of recent work and develops the author's views of what autonomy means in the real world. The author writes with passion and concern about his topic, combining a scholarly, phenomen-ological approach to ethics and personal identity with an awareness of the needs of vulnerable older people and their carers. The book will have wide appeal among bioethicists and health care professionals.

George J. Agich is the F.J. O'Neill Chair in Clinical Bioethics and Chairman of the Department of Bioethics at the Cleveland Clinic Foundation, Professor of Clinical Medicine at Ohio State University, and Adjunct Professor of Philosophy at Bowling Green State University. His previous books are *Responsibility in Health Care* (1982), and *The Price of Health* (1986), and he is a member of the editorial board of *The American Journal of Bioethics* and other journals.

Dependence and Autonomy in Old Age

An Ethical Framework for Long-Term Care

Second and Revised Edition

George J. Agich

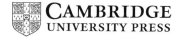
CAMBRIDGE
UNIVERSITY PRESS

PUBLISHED BY THE PRESS SYNDICATE OF THE UNIVERSITY OF CAMBRIDGE
The Pitt Building, Trumpington Street, Cambridge, United Kingdom

CAMBRIDGE UNIVERSITY PRESS
The Edinburgh Building, Cambridge CB2 2RU, UK
40 West 20th Street, New York, NY 10011–4211, USA
477 Williamstown Road, Port Melbourne, VIC 3207, Australia
Ruiz de Alarcón 13, 28014 Madrid, Spain
Dock House, The Waterfront, Cape Town 8001, South Africa

http://www.cambridge.org

First published 2003

Printed in the United Kingdom at the University Press, Cambridge

Typefaces Minion 10/12 pt. and Dax   *System* LaTeX 2$_\varepsilon$ [TB]

A catalog record for this book is available from the British Library

Library of Congress Cataloging-in-Publication data
Agich, George J., 1947 –
Dependence and autonomy in old age : an ethical framework for long-term care /
George J. Agich. – 2nd edn., rev.
       p.   cm.
Previously published as: Autonomy and long-term care.
Includes bibliographical references and index.
ISBN 0 521 00920 0 (paperback)
1. Aged – Long-term care – Moral and ethical aspects.   2. Autonomy (Psychology) in old age.
3. Autonomy (Philosophy)   I. Agich, George J., 1947 – Autonomy and long-term care.   II. Title.
RC954.3 .A44 2003
174′.2–dc21   2002031406

ISBN 0 521 00920 0 paperback

Contents

Preface

After receiving numerous queries about a paperback edition for classroom and other use, I undertook revisions to *Autonomy and Long-Term Care*, the predecessor of this edition, with the intention of bringing my ideas about autonomy in old age to a larger audience. Oxford University Press, publisher of the original book, ultimately decided against a second edition. Fortunately, an arrangement with Cambridge University Press was worked out that permitted the publication of this revised edition. Dr Richard Barling, Medical Publishing Director of Cambridge University Press, has been incredibly supportive of this project as discussions with OUP proceeded. Jeffrey House and Edith Barry of OUP were also very helpful throughout these discussions and I am very grateful for their longstanding good will.

Work on this edition was supported with research help provided through the F.J. O'Neill Chair in Clinical Bioethics. The longstanding support of Nancy O'Neill, Hugh O'Neill, and the F.J. O'Neill Charitable Foundation for Bioethics at the Cleveland Clinic Foundation has been truly remarkable. Their continued support during my tenure in the O'Neill Chair has been outstanding and gratefully appreciated.

The first edition of this book was dedicated to my mother-in-law and father-in-law. My father-in-law had been diagnosed with Alzheimer's disease and required institutional care, so their view of the problems discussed therein was far more significantly 'inside' than my own. Several years ago, my own mother also developed memory loss and confusion that eventually necessitated her moving into an assisted-living center, where she resided until her death. These events are deeply personal reminders that the challenges of respecting the autonomy of disabled elders are often bound up with family relationships, commitments, and emotional meanings that must be accommodated in ethical analysis. Attention to autonomy in long-term care is thus important less for philosophical reasons than for the existential impact that disabilities create for persons who deserve our love and respect. I hope that this work challenges and helps caregivers to reexamine their commitments and practices to enhance the dimming autonomy of old people and the threatened autonomy of disabled individuals.

The primary examples used in this revision, as in the original work, are frail and disabled elders. The problems associated with long-term care apply to a much wider range of chronic conditions, not all of them debilitating or end-of-life. I have dealt with some of these areas in papers written after the first edition was published: for example, the meaning of actual autonomy and long-term care in the context of chronic disease (Agich 1995a, 1995b), schizophrenia (Agich 1997), consent in research on Alzheimer's disease (Agich 1996), and the meaning of autonomy in Alzheimer's disease and dementia (Agich 1994, 1999). Others have adapted the concept of actual autonomy in empirical studies of rehabilitation (Proot et al. 1998, 2000a, 2000b, 2000c). To avoid compromising the line of argument, however, I chose not to introduce these kinds of examples in any significant way, for fear of losing focus. This omission is justified primarily because the application of the concept of actual autonomy in contexts like rehabilitation tends to confirm, rather than challenge or compromise, the main lines of my analysis of autonomy in old age.

My work on the problem of autonomy and long-term care began in 1987 when I first addressed some of the difficulties associated with its meaning and function. I saw the need for an alternative to the mainstream, liberal view of autonomy as applied to the complex clinical problems and settings of old age. A viable alternative should preserve the core commitments of liberal theory, so I avoided seeking refuge from the problems of respecting autonomy in communitarian or care ethics, even though the approaches are compatible with my own. Instead, I wanted to develop a more nuanced concept of autonomy that was more appropriate to the concrete reality of the long-term care context.

I have had little interest in cataloging the range of ethical problems in nursing homes and to some extent I have avoided directly confronting a number of important societal problems involving the aging of the population, such as the allocation of resources or intergenerational issues of justice. This work, instead, is an extended essay on the practical meaning and function of autonomy under the conditions of disability that create the need for chronic care. Its guiding idea is that autonomy is a central ethical concept in this context, but only if it can be refurbished. The argument is developed along two lines: first, an extended appraisal of the liberal view of autonomy and its applicability in long-term care and, second, a phenomenological exposition of the meaning of actual autonomy in the everyday world and in long-term care. The goal of the phenomenological account of actual autonomy is to set out a framework within which practical work on autonomy and long-term care can proceed. The analysis and discussion are at certain points rather coarse grained, because the objective of this book is programmatic, namely, to set out a framework for practical thinking about autonomy in the context of long-term care. This book does not purport to address fully the range of ethical issues associated with geriatrics and gerontology. The ethical theory in the book is not fully developed or justified to any serious extent and there is little in the way of prescriptions or normative rules to guide conduct. Instead, I have aimed to develop a framework for rethinking and reconsidering the everyday ethics of long-term care. I accept that ethical conflict, dilemma, and tragedy are inescapable features of this setting, and I do not think that theoretical analysis is the right tool to achieve the practical objectives of improving the quality of care. I strongly believe that well-motivated caregivers can improve their practices if they could be provided with a useful way to think about respecting the autonomy of persons needing long-term care. For such a framework to have practical significance, readers will need to adopt its vantage point to inform their thinking and action. The book is thus motivated by the belief that prescriptive advice is far less useful than a fresh presentation of the complex reality of autonomy to reveal its manifestations in the sometimes cold and comfortless confines of long-term care. I have the confidence that those who are situated closer to the phenomena of old age and disability are better able to devise solutions to problems or to make improvements in programs than someone trained in bioethics and philosophy.

The analysis of actual autonomy, social action, and the world of everyday life that occupies Chapters 4 and 5 has deep roots in phenomenology. Sources for this analysis were diverse, ranging from philosophical phenomenological work to concrete existential and sociological studies. I have chosen to spare the reader much of the theoretical and methodological detail of phenomenological philosophy, because phenomenological approaches often expire on the doorstep with detailed discussions of method that obstruct a passage to the very phenomena they tout. This work is guided by the conviction that adhering to the phenomenological battle cry *to the things themselves* is best accomplished by keeping attention fixed on the phenomena in question. The ethical and practical significance of autonomy ultimately rests on its presence in the world of everyday life. Thus, pointing out autonomy's least well-known features seemed more important than discussing the methodological processes by which these features are made apparent. This work owes much to philosophical phenomenology as well as to the ethnographic work inspired by Alfred Schutz's program of a phenomenology of the social world (1967). If actual autonomy does provide a viable focus for ethical reflection, then perhaps this work will inspire bioethicists to give the phenomenology of the world of everyday life far greater attention in addressing problems in clinical ethics. This book is best regarded as a work on how to plan and conduct a visit to a new country rather than as a detailed travel guide. It sets out a framework for improving the care of elders in long-term care by highlighting the actual ways that autonomy is manifested by individuals needing chronic care.

Work on the present edition was facilitated by outstanding preparatory work done by Candice Kieffer, with the assistance of Barbara Workman, who scanned the first edition to provide a reliable basis for revision and transcribed my numerous attempts to express a point or develop an argument. Ray Klancar cheerfully tracked down many references and performed a yeoman's task in proofreading the entire manuscript. Finally, Nate Stewart provided an updated review of recent philosophical work on autonomy. I am grateful for their dedicated help and to the many colleagues and audiences who have discussed my ideas about autonomy and long-term care over the last decade.

G.J.A.
Shaker Heights, Ohio
April 2002

Introduction

Autonomy and long-term care are a remarkably paradoxical conjunction. Individuals need long-term care because they suffer illnesses and incapacities that compromise their ability to function independently or to choose rationally. Yet the standard concept of autonomy in bioethics stresses the ideals of independence and rational free choice, ideals that appear ephemeral in the face of the wide range of impairments that cause individuals to need long-term care. No doubt such individuals are vulnerable and so might benefit from the protection afforded by various autonomy-derived rights such as noninterference. The paradox is that the underlying concept of autonomy involves a view of persons as robust and independent, whereas the reality of long-term care shows individuals who need support and companionship, needs that seem inimical to this ideal. The paradox thus involves the contrast between capacities central to standard views of autonomy and the actual capacities of individuals who need long-term care: independence versus dependence and capacities associated with agency versus functional frailties. The paradox arises when the fragility and vulnerability of individuals needing long-term care are approached from the perspective of the standard view of autonomy that implicitly involves a robust concept of individual capacity.

The standard view of autonomy is a product of the deep and variegated liberal tradition of thought that is at the foundation of contemporary democracy and bioethical thought. In this view, autonomy is primarily a phenomenon involving independence of action, speech, and thought. It provides the broad foundation for a wide range of political, legal, civil, and human rights and the philosophical basis on which individuals can resist the coercive interference of external authorities or powers in their lives.

The ideals implicit in this concept of autonomy include independence and self-determination, the ability to make rational and free decisions, and an ability to accurately assess what constitutes the individual's own best interest. This concept of autonomy has led to worries about paternalism, the use of (varying degrees of) coercion to impose another's vision – where the other might be the state, private institutions, or individuals – on a single individual or class of individuals. The concept of autonomy so understood supports a set of values such as independence and self-determination that have provided the normative standards around which tyranny, oppression, and even the benevolent use of power over vulnerable individuals have been opposed.

If we approach the task of enhancing the autonomy of elders in long-term care from a critical appreciation of this tradition, an occlusion becomes obvious that requires attention. Autonomy and long-term care are each rather diffuse cultural ideas. This is so much the case that it is difficult to pierce through the cultural and ideological aura that surrounds these terms. To realistically reassess the meaning and function of autonomy in long-term care, then, requires that we pay attention to the symbolic meanings of autonomy and long-term care, because these meanings not only set the context or stage for the analysis, but also complicate its execution.

Long-term care images

The term *long-term care* conjures up many images; few of them are felicitous. Long-term care seems to hang like a pall covering the inevitable coffin that awaits us all. Surprisingly, in our culture it is less death than long-term care that strikes us as so repugnant. This reaction may represent a profound psychological defense against death, to be sure, but its immediate effect is to place long-term care center stage in an unfavorable light. The images of long-term care are images of frailty and despair, loneliness and destitution, and above all a profound sense of loss, a loss not only of things, but of who and what we are. These attitudes undoubtedly reflect society's perceptions of the institutions that are often thought to be the main providers of long-term care, namely, nursing homes. Anthropologists and sociologists regard nursing homes as anything but humane (Gubrium 1975; Henry 1963; Kayser-Jones 1981; Laird 1979; Lidz, Fischer, and Arnold 1990; O'Brien 1989; Savishinsky 1991; Shield 1988; Vesperi 1983, Watson and Maxwell 1977). They are frequently seen as places of exploitation (of staff as well as of residents). They stimulate either moral outrage or revulsion. These reactions are shaped by latent image: a blabbering, incoherent, disheveled elder strapped into a geri-chair, withdrawn or beckoning for attention, but invariably ignored by staff who, without emotion, expression, or enthusiasm, perfunctorily perform the onerous tasks of daily bed and body work that are made even more difficult by the niggling demands of residents. The image is coupled with the olfactory assault of urine, excrement, and myriad other unpleasant odors that suffuse drab corridors or insipid sitting rooms where residents sit transfixed, each in his or her own world. There are also disturbing sounds of people moaning from down the hall, crying out, one elder scolding another harshly, others weeping in protest. No wonder that the pall of long-term care is as feared as the coffin it covers! Long-term care seems suffused with a terrifying absence, the absence of a meaningful sense of control, dignity, or identity. It is an appalling state of living death, somewhere just this side of madness.

Like many taken-for-granted beliefs, the nursing home-dominated image of long-term care is in its general form brutally apt, but it harbors latent meanings that require careful exegesis and qualification. For one thing, not all long-term care is institutional. Despite perceptions to the contrary, only 4.3 percent of those over the age of 65 live in institutions, a percentage that rises dramatically with age, ranging from 1.1 percent for those aged 65–74 years to 4.5 percent for those aged 75–84 years and 19 percent for those aged 85 and above (Administration on Aging 2000). Twenty-five percent of those in institutions will spend at least 12 months there, and at least 10 percent will be patients for 5 years or more (Kemper and Murtaugh 1991: 597). The chance of being in a geriatric facility significantly increases with age.

The confluence of several macro trends in developed countries – older population age structures, higher incidence of noncommunicable disease, lowered fertility, increased geographical mobility, and the rapid advance in medical technology – has led to a steep rise in numbers of institutionalized elderly. (Kinsella and Velkoff 2001: 69).

Cross-national comparisons of living arrangements of elders lead to three conclusions: women in developed countries are more likely than men to live alone as they age; generally both elderly men and women in developing countries live with adult children; and the use of institutions to care for frail elders varies widely around the world (Kinsella and Velkoff 2001: 65). In the United States, approximately 22 percent of the elderly population will spend some time in an institution after they reach the age of 85 (Siegel and Taeuber 1986: 101), but 'the fact remains that relatively small proportions of elderly populations reside in institutions at any given time' (Kinsella and Velkoff 2001: 69). Most elders do not live in nursing homes, but remain in contact with their families and friends (Shanas 1979). In 1998, 67 percent of older non-institutionalized persons in the United States lived in a family setting (Administration on Aging 2000). Even for institutionalized elders, dozens of individuals outside the institution, including family, friends, neighbors, clergy, social workers, lawyers, and doctors, will be involved in their care and directly touched by their fate (Savishinsky 1991: 9–10).

Family, friends, or in-home services thus deliver a considerable amount of care in the home. Such care involves help with the tasks of daily living ranging from personal assistance and services such as food preparation, hygiene, administration of medication, to companionship, assistance in shopping, and entertainment. Indeed, discussions of long-term care frequently presume that the nursing home is the natural locus of long-term care, whereas it is actually a member of a heterogeneous class of services. Although the nursing home paradigm distorts our understanding of the reality and issues associated with long-term care, its prominence indicates something quite significant about our latent cultural expectations and anxieties.

In reality there are, at least, two kinds of nursing homes (sometimes existing within the same physical structure): the so-called skilled nursing home and the institution that provides only intermediate care (Lidz, Fischer, and Arnold 1990). The distinction in kind makes an important practical difference. In the United States, Medicare pays only for skilled nursing care, as does most private insurance. Medicare-paid nursing care is designed to aid the transition from hospital for elders who have suffered an acute health crisis. It is short term and rehabilitation oriented. There are strict time, disease, and dollar limits (Diamond 1986: 1288). Although Medicare is the only real national long-term care program in existence in the United States, it is remarkably short-term oriented. Medicaid pays for nursing home care only after a patient has become indigent. As a social safety net, it is situated frightfully near the ground. No wonder elders (and their families) perceive its support with such apprehension, for it means a fall, sometimes a precipitously long fall, from economic sufficiency to indigence. This economic fact adds to the perception of long-term care as involving a loss of independence. This situation is not confined to the United States. Reiner Leidel (1995: 50) reports that old-age dependency has been rising during the last 20 years in almost all 12 states of the European Union. Elders who are declining in health and ability to care for themselves understandably live in apprehension of the economic (as well as psychological and social) consequences of their fall. This point is driven home by the data on disability in old age:

In 1994–95 more than half of the older population (52.5%) reported having at least one disability. One-third has at least one severe disability. Over 4.4 million (14%) had difficulty in carrying out activities of daily living (ADLs) and 6.5 million (21%) reported difficulties with instrumental activities of daily living (IADLs). The percentages with disabilities increase sharply with age (Administration on Aging 2000: 11).

At the same time, Kinsella and Velkoff report that: 'Recent data and rigorous analysis strongly suggest that rates of disability in a number of developed countries are declining' (2001: 41). When disability strikes, the cost of medical care can drive elders toward becomingly paupers (Diamond 1986: 1289). Destitution is the norm for those individuals who are cut off from the discretionary income that in Western societies is the almost universal measure of social status and worth. This point applies equally to those who have recently fallen from economic grace, as well as to those who have always depended on public aid, because discretion over the use of even limited funds is as important for the poor as for the middle class or wealthy.

The everyday reality of the nursing home is thus strikingly dissonant with the competing popular image of retirement as a stable life filled with fulfilling leisure activities. Long-term care represents a state of economical, psychological, and social instability. It is little wonder that long-term care encourages rhetorical appeals to autonomy. Autonomy in long-term care is a slogan employed for the liberation of the frail and destitute old. Increasing autonomy in long-term care is bioethics response to the complex cultural crisis that disability and aging represent. Like many slogans, it needs careful analysis if it is to promote any practically effective and ethically defensible reforms. Understanding the cultural meaning of the nursing home as the symbolic setting for long-term care can help us to understand both the attraction and limitation of the appeal to autonomy as a central ethical concern and principle for long-term care.

Given our cultural revulsion to the sometimes brutal and stark reality of nursing home life, appealing to considerations of autonomy both salves our sense of moral outrage and yet preserves the distance that we so dearly want to maintain between ourselves and the idea of loss and incapacity that figuratively oozes from the image. Autonomy is attractive because it provides a ready-made vernacular of rights that seem to capture what at first glance bothers us about long-term care, namely, the effacement of autonomy and functional capacity, expressed in the pronounced dependence of nursing home existence.

Nursing homes are examples of what Erving Goffman termed total institutions (Goffman 1960, 1961). Like army barracks, mental hospitals, nunneries, and prisons, nursing homes are *total* in the sense that they isolate, control, and reconstitute the daily lives of their residents. Stripping away and reconstituting the identities of their residents through rituals of initiation and degradation accomplish this. They require the participation of the residents in certain kinds of prerequisite activities and behaviors for gaining privileges that we often take for granted as everyday liberties. Opposition to total institutions is a well-known theme in democratic social thought. Ironically, the consequence of the most committed criticism of such institutions is not always ideal as the case of the deinstitutionalization of the mentally ill shows. Panaceas, appealing as they seem in theory and as powerfully as they perform in rhetoric, seldom work in practice. In the case of severely debilitated elders, it is paradoxical to acknowledge the need for institutional care and to regard the oppressive locus of such care as reformable by a large injection of liberal values.

The pivot of talk of liberalizing nursing home care is the concept of autonomy. It is manifested in numerous well-intentioned proposals, such as insisting on full-disclosure preadmission agreements, creation of patient ombudsmen or nursing home ethics committees, insisting on delineation of a basic set of resident rights, or establishment of detailed values histories for each resident (Hofland 1990). Collectively, these approaches attend to what bothers us most about the surface reality of nursing home existence, yet saves us from having to deal with the messy deep reality of being old and frail. It saves us from confronting the economic, physical, psychological, and social conditions that engender nursing home care and the more difficult ethical questions that the daily care of individuals requiring long-term care poses.

Autonomy

Like long-term care, autonomy involves a diffuse set of meanings that are culturally as well as philosophically determined. It would thus be a mistake to assume that the term *autonomy* has a consistent meaning or usage in ethical theory, political theory, or everyday contexts. Recent philosophical work on autonomy has included a discussion of a range of concerns that generally tends to avoid use of the term itself (Christman 1988, 1989). Autonomy refers to a broad set of qualities that are generally, though not universally, regarded with approval. Autonomy is taken to be equivalent to liberty, either positive or negative liberty in Isaiah Berlin's sense (1969: 118–72), self-rule, self-determination, freedom of will, dignity, integrity, individuality, independence, responsibility, and self-knowledge; it is also identified with the qualities of self-assertion, critical reflection, freedom from obligation, absence of external causation, and knowledge of one's own interest, and is related to actions, beliefs, reasons for acting, rules, the will of others, thoughts, as well as principles (Beauchamp and Childress 1983; Dworkin 1978, 1988; Gilbert 2000). Treatment of autonomy in the gerontological bioethics literature has a similar wide range of meanings (Thomasma 1984) involving a diverse set of tensions or polarities (Collopy 1986, 1988) that suggests that respecting autonomy is likely to be far more complex than is apparent at first glance (Donchin 2000).

This wide range of usage suggests that it is unlikely that an essential or core meaning underlies these various employments; therefore, it would be futile to try to develop an essential definition of autonomy as a starting point for practical ethical analysis of long-term care. Rather than arguing for a core or essential definition of autonomy, it would be best to acknowledge that the meaning of autonomy is irremediably context dependent. It would be wrong to conclude that these observations imply that the meaning of the concept is so relative that meaningful philosophical treatment is precluded. Certainly, some accounts of autonomy will fail because they try to force the concept to accomplish what it is incapable of achieving in certain contexts of concern. An adequate philosophical treatment of autonomy in long-term care must come to terms with the contextual nature of the concept of autonomy instead of relying on abstract, theoretically provided definitions. This point implies that the concept of autonomy in long-term care must be shaped with a clear vision of the practical purposes that autonomy might serve in the context of long-term care itself.

Autonomy, however, is not only an important philosophical concept; it is a significant cultural ideal. In the guise of independence, it has been a perennial feature of American society. In the early days of the Republic, Alexis de Tocqueville noted the peculiar tendency of Americans to draw apart and to keep to themselves: 'Each citizen is disposed to isolate himself from the mass of his fellows and to draw apart with his family and friends. It not only makes each man forget his forefathers, but it conceals him from his descendants and separates him from his contemporaries' (quoted in Christiansen 1983: 35). More recently, American society has been characterized as the *lonely crowd* (Riesman 1950) and as engaged in a collective pursuit of loneliness (Slater 1970). Indeed, some authors have noted that the concept of individual freedom held by elderly Americans and their families rests on a sweeping faith and confidence of the individual in his own competence and mastery, which, in turn, produces a definition of personal identity predicated on independence and self-reliance (Clark 1971: 265). This cultural ideal results in a variety of secondary defenses against dependence: a denial of need, hostility toward helpers even in the face of disabilities and limitations that require assistance from others, contempt for the real or imagined weakness of others, and, in some cases, an inflated self-image. The cultural attitude that constitutes an aversion for dependence has been termed *counterdependence* (Christiansen 1983: 52–128; Rogers 1974).

The attitude of counterdependence assumes that any form of dependence is tantamount to a degrading submission. This view is understandable given the dominance of the concept of autonomy as negative freedom, namely, the idea that individual freedom consists fundamentally in the noninterference of others in the life of the individual. The over-determination of negative freedom is partly due to its association in Anglo-American political and ethical theory with a set of beliefs about individual freedom that prominently includes self-reliance, personal preference, and self-assertion. (Christiansen 1983: 41–4)

Self-reliance refers to the capacity to provide for one's own needs. In the course of aging, however, dependence begins as the diminishment of one's powers of self-reliance. The problem is not with self-reliance as such, but rather that self-reliance defines individual worth. Lacking the ability to be self-reliant contributes to the feeling of worthlessness experienced by many old people. If identity and value are grounded in one's ability to be self-supporting, then physical infirmity and disability can compromise one's sense of personal worth precisely by compromising self-reliance. This point is admirably summarized in the notion of active life expectancy as an empirical measure of population health. This measure involves activities and abilities such as bathing, dressing, transfer or mobility, and eating that are correlated with a sense of functional well-being; loss of these functional abilities represents loss of independence (Katz et al. 1983).

A second concept associated with the idea of individual freedom is personal preference. Personal preference focuses discussion of autonomy on the phenomena of choice and decision. Indeed, choice is of such importance that attention to one's wishes, desires, and impulses comprises a significant set of concerns in the ethical analysis of human action. This focus, however, makes it difficult, if not impossible, to question whether the values implied by one's desires, impulses, or wishes are worth having. From the fact that I choose something on the basis of my desire, for example a certain kind of food, it does not follow that that something is good for me. Attention to my wants or preferences, however, not only renders the question of the good of the objects of choice irrelevant, it restricts the domain of ethics to but one feature among many defining human moral agency. Choice is undeniably important, but not all-important. Attention to the phenomena of choice and decision making has had the unfortunate consequence of rendering otiose other features of autonomy.

Third, the concept of individual freedom includes the value of self-assertion as a basic requirement, namely, that one actively pursues the fulfillment of one's desires. It is not enough to have desires or to make choices; one must be actively engaged in their fulfillment or accomplishment. So construed, autonomy commits individuals to a seemingly ceaseless pursuit of the fulfillment of their preferences, for without such fulfillment autonomy itself is seen as useless or empty. Whatever thwarts the attainment of one's desires is seen as curtailing freedom; hence, noninterference becomes the obvious imperative under this concept of autonomy. It is commonly admitted, however, that this view is odd and even destructive when applied to children, yet the restraint or mastery of desire that is characteristic of maturation seems to be regarded somehow as inappropriate or wrong in the case of adults! A moment's reflection should indicate that this is a fundamental mistake. Acquiring any sort of skill or expertise, whether as a child or adult, involves discipline of unruly tendencies or desires. Learning always involves a subordination of the immediate fulfillment of desire to wider ends and purposes.

Autonomy and long-term care: the problem

The dissonance between the image of the robust, striving, and unencumbered individual making her own way competently in the world and even the most banal limitations that underlie the need for long-term care should be readily apparent. Some adult individuals, for example frail elders, are generally not fully self-reliant; they often lack the psychological ability, physical energy, or social and economic prerequisites necessary to pursue their preferences. The view of autonomy that takes as a defining feature the pursuit of all preferences – just because those preferences are preferences of the individual – seems to foredoom as paternalistic and objectionable any attempt to respond to an elder's evident need. Where desire reigns, need recedes. Thus, the diminished capacity that brings elders into long-term care contributes to the view that dependence entails subservience and inferiority; but if independence is only, or primarily, valued, then we should not be surprised to find that responding even to basic human needs is fraught with contradiction.

Addressing the conjunction of autonomy and long-term care thus presents two types of problems at two different levels: first, the level of concepts involving the meaning of long-term care and the meaning of autonomy and, second, the practical difficulties associated with actual autonomy and the reality of long-term care. These four elements interplay in a complex pattern.

The most striking feature of long-term care is that adult individuals suffering from diseases and illnesses of being old experience a compromised vigor and ability to function that requires regular care ranging from help in the activities of daily living, such as housework, food preparation, and hygiene, to highly skilled nursing and medical care. Functional disabilities that frequently bring with them vulnerabilities define elders as a class of individuals requiring long-term care. Because elders requiring long-term care often deviate in obvious ways from the ideal of the competent, rational, and free decision maker that is implicit in the commonplace understanding of autonomy, various mechanisms have been devised to protect elders from unwarranted intrusion. These mechanisms include the use of various legal advocacy and guardianship measures to endow elders with specific rights as well as the use of surrogate decision-making procedures, especially in the case of refusal of life-sustaining medical care. Reliance on surrogate decision making is an interesting development in long-term care, primarily growing out of the acute care context (Buchanan and Brock 1989). The reality of long-term care apparently forces even the staunchest proponent of autonomy as independence to deal with the reality of an impaired decision-making capacity or incompetence that is an ineliminable feature of long-term care.

This response is both understandable and troubling. It is understandable because the reality is such that elderly individuals who require long-term care frequently experience various physical, psychological, and social disabilities and deprivations that should give us pause. These frailties suggest that the ideal of the person that underlies the standard view of autonomy is inapplicable in many of these cases or simply fails to provide much practical assistance for either restoring or sustaining the degree and kind of autonomy that is present. Primarily because it is dominated by an abstract and ideal concept of the autonomous individual that fails to jibe with the reality of long-term care, the concept of autonomy as independence simply proves inadequate and has to be refurbished if it is to function importantly in the context of long-term care.

These observations point to the second problem that arises if we critically reflect on the applicability and usefulness of commonplace understandings of autonomy in long-term care, namely, the nature of autonomy itself. The traditional liberal view of autonomy tends to direct attention to specific problems associated with decision making. This view is not surprising given the powerful place that the related concepts of independence, self-determination, and rights enjoy in our culture. These concepts, embodied in the Anglo-American legal system, exert a significant influence on bioethical thinking. Hence, autonomy has come to be defined primarily in terms of a concept of human persons as rational, independent agents and decision makers, who are assumed to be competent and who can be understood without serious reference to society or history.

Independent decision makers are insulated by a fabric of rights that protects them from the intrusive and coercive influence of the state or other individuals. Indeed, the individual is often seen as standing in opposition to society or the state that is assumed to pose a threat to the integrity of the self. Individuals are idealized in such a way that the expression of uniquely individual beliefs and values is given primacy over other goods or values. Furthermore, decision making is regarded as a rational process that can be understood or explained in terms of decision theory; communicative interactions between individuals are thought to involve primarily the exchange of information as evidenced by the stress on disclosure of information in the legal doctrine of informed consent. This view of autonomy is remarkably abstract and assumes an ideal view of persons. It is not only deficient as a general theory of the meaning of actual autonomy, but, more pointedly, is not well suited for conceptualizing the ethical problems associated with long-term care. For this reason, the concept of autonomy itself must be reassessed and revamped if it is to play a significant role in theoretically and practically clarifying the ethics of long-term care.

The assumptions and implications of the commonplace understanding of autonomy as independence orient reflection on long-term care to relatively dramatic conflicts expressible in terms of rights. As a consequence, more mundane day-to-day experiences and encounters of elders with caregivers in long-term care tend to be overlooked, in part because they lack the conflictual, dramatic, and discrete characteristics required by the standard view. A truly helpful ethics of long-term care, however, would incorporate a concept of autonomy that is interstitial to the typical everyday reality of long-term care, not one that fixates on the unusual or atypical. The context from which the main concept of autonomy comes is the political/legal realm; it is further supported by the reality of acute care medicine that hand-in-glove seems to support a concept of ethics that is problem or issue based. Unfortunately, political/legal treatments of autonomy typically marginalize questions of relationship, quality of care, and the affective dimension of clinical encounters, concerns that are significant in long-term care as well.

The common view that autonomy is tantamount to independence has important implications for long-term care. First, the cultural dominance of this model of autonomy creates a backlash against dependence of any sort, so that the frail and infirm old who require long-term care are especially vulnerable to the pejorative meanings associated with dependence. They are seen and frequently see themselves as burdensome and less than full persons. As a class, these elders are treated as deviants from the images of robustly active retirement for which the oxymoron *active retirement* has become a battle cry.

Second, autonomy as independence injects a predominantly adversarial and conflictual set of metaphors into thinking about long-term care. Like so much discourse in our society, the language of rights eclipses other ethical language. As a result, long-term care is mainly thought of in terms of problems that can or should be dealt with by establishing legal rights or promulgating regulations. The goal of these efforts is to force caregivers to conform to the standards of a liberal polity and respect the rights of their wards. Ironically, when elders lose the abilities assumed to be present for autonomy as independence, society is less enthusiastically committed to dealing with the aftermath. Frail and sick elders are infantilized by social institutions and programs that afford them entitlements to *services*, but under conditions that hide them from public view.

Third, the asymmetry between autonomy as negative freedom (the vision of the agent as independent and rationally competent) and the economic, physical, psychological, and social needs of elders propelled into long-term care forces to prominence the question 'Is autonomy really the central value and concept for thinking about the ethics of long-term care?' It is if it can be phenomenologically re-interpreted to sustain an ethically robust framework for the practice of long-term care.

The goal of this work is to articulate just such a framework. Without rejecting the central commitments of the liberal view of autonomy, I propose a complementary framework to open the everyday reality of long-term care to ethical analysis. This alternative framework develops a view of the nature of *actual* autonomy predicated on a concrete understanding of the everyday experience of autonomy in long-term care. This framework involves a shift of attention from autonomy as independence to the concrete manifestations of autonomy in the everyday world of life. The framework involves a developmentally oriented and phenomenologically derived account of the ordinary or everyday sense of autonomy in terms of concrete human action in the shared world of social life. The framework brings into focus the full range of caregiving interactions as well as the structure of caregiving relationships. It opens up the complex reality of the long-term care of elders for clinical ethical reflection.

2

The liberal theory of autonomy

Autonomy is a touchstone for much analysis and discussion in the field of bioethics. To understand its proper application in the context of long-term care, it is important to appreciate the lineage and limitations of this concept by considering its roots in the liberal theory of autonomy. Although there are significant limitations associated with the liberal theory of autonomy, most of these limitations are tractable. Liberal theory is not itself the problem, but the extension of what is primarily a political and legal theory into ethics levels the complex landscape of moral life. We need not reject liberal theory, but can confine it within its proper borders and we can supplement its contribution to ethical analysis and practice by offering a fuller and more adequate view of what it means to be an autonomous agent. Pursuing these points can entangle us in the wider debate over the modern, liberal view of the self and the political and ethical commitments of this view involving a set of controversies that are remote from the subject of this book. For this reason, this book contains only a limited allusion to this complex debate. The goal is to develop an account of autonomy compatible with liberal theory that establishes the practical utility of autonomy for the ethical analysis of long-term care. To do so, the concept of autonomy is examined in a concrete and practical way to establish a framework for re-thinking the ethics of long-term care.

Although the liberal theory affords an inadequate vantage point from which to survey the ethics of providing long-term care for impaired elders, its weaknesses do not require that autonomy be displaced in favor of other principles or values, such as care, community, or tradition. To be sure, these values have a place in a treatment of the ethics of long-term care, but they are best regarded as aspects of a fuller understanding of the meaning of human autonomy rather than as independent principles.

Taking the liberal theory of autonomy as a starting point, I argue that it should be restricted to the political/legal realm. This restriction clears the field for development of an alternative treatment of autonomy in subsequent chapters, a treatment that is far more conducive to the realities of long-term care than is the liberal view. In the course of the present chapter, I discuss the communitarian critique of liberalism and argue that communitarianism and liberal theory share questionable assumptions about the nature of justification in ethics. I defend a contextualist alternative, which has practical implications for the analysis of autonomy in the context of long-term care. Finally, I argue that the language of rights, the common vernacular of liberalism, does have an important, but circumscribed, role in long-term care. Paternalism, the *bête noire* of liberal theory, is often regarded as the dominant constraint on a contextual treatment of autonomy, like that of autonomy in long-term care. I argue that the critique of paternalism has obscured the viability of a parentalist approach to provide a viable alternative in terms of which to construct an ethics of caring for frail and dependent elders.

Pluralism, toleration, and neutrality

Autonomy is a central value in American society; it gives expression to a basic set of legal and political ideals that have gone under the name of liberalism. Central to political liberalism is the idea of individual freedom or autonomy. The term *autonomy* refers to a broad set of qualities that are generally, though not universally, regarded with approval in Western societies. Central to its treatment in political contexts is the concept of independence or what has been termed *negative freedom*, the freedom to be left alone (Berlin 1969). Implicit in this negative concept, to be sure, is a positive concept involving qualities of self-assertion, critical reflection, absence of external causation, and knowledge of one's own interest qualities that are themselves indeterminately related to concepts of actions, beliefs, and reasons for acting (Dworkin 1988). The mainstream treatments of autonomy, however, usually have little to say about the positive characteristics or capacities that are required for negative freedom and are content instead to worry about the kind of social arrangements that interfere with the exercise of individual freedom of action or choice (Young 1986). These treatments are expressive of deep-seated cultural values that comprise the conceptual context for my examination of autonomy and long-term care.

As a cultural ideal, autonomy usually involves a vision of individuals freely living their lives according to their own beliefs and values, with minimal interference by the state or others. Minimal involvement or intrusion of the state is permitted, for example, to regulate and secure public safety because of the belief that such involvement ultimately promotes or permits individual freedom of action. In things that matter most, however, other individuals and the state should have no say. Indeed, implicit in the cultural value of autonomy is a deep suspicion about shared beliefs and values. Things are valuable, because autonomous individuals value them. Along with skepticism over external authority is a deep-seated relativism about values and the moral good.

Given the stress on individuality and skepticism about beliefs and values that do not happen to be one's own – I leave the meaning of this crucial phrase unexamined as it typically is in the context under discussion – proponents of the liberal theory defend two further concepts, namely, pluralism and toleration, as unavoidable corollaries of autonomy. Pluralism is the view that there are many viable concepts of the good life, many viable concepts of how one's life should be conducted. These concepts are neither different versions of a single homogeneous good nor related in any discernible hierarchical pattern. Thus, difference is unavoidable and ineliminable. Because of difference, conflicts and disagreement unavoidably arise in the course of daily living. For this reason, toleration is an essential corollary of pluralism. Because we can expect that even reasonable persons will disagree about fundamental values and concepts of the good life, practical acceptance of the views of others – views that we may find wrongheaded, objectionable, or even repulsive – is required. Since liberals accept that we may live with those who do not share our own ideals or else succumb to interminable conflict or resort to force to settle disagreement, toleration is the logical requirement.

Given that diversity of viewpoints (pluralism) and disagreement among reasonable persons have become features of modern life and medical practice, political liberalism is the doctrine that the state should be neutral with respect to such disputes. An action or decision will count as neutral only if its justification does not appeal to some presumed intrinsic superiority of its own concept of the good life. Neutrality understood in this procedural fashion thus is silent on the specific goals that the liberal society ought to pursue. This does not necessarily mean that neutrality requires a so-called minimal state, that is, a state that, for the most part, renounces substantive commitments that embody the content of any particular vision of the good, even though libertarians frequently assume just such a conclusion (Nozick 1974).

Liberals need not deny that freedom could or should mean more than the absence of governmental interference in nonpolitical areas (Larmore 1987: 47). It would be consistent, though rare, for an avowed liberal to defend substantive ideals of (positive) freedom, including, for example, ideals of self-realization or the provision of meaningful choices. These positive ideals, however, could be defended on ethical grounds. Because political neutrality need not be absolute, other substantive moral commitments are possible, even required, on a liberal perspective. Indeed, the liberal advocacy of negative freedom occurs most forcefully when particular ideas of the good life or ideals of positive autonomy are pressed on unwilling persons in the public and political realm. The rights to consent to and to refuse treatment are well-known examples of the application of the principle of noninterference to health care. Such rights protect vulnerable patients from the authority and power of health professionals and institutions alike.

The ideal of neutrality requires that the state should not promote any particular concept of the good life because of its presumed intrinsic superiority. This neutrality is not a neutrality of outcome but of procedure. Some visions of the good life may, in fact, be supported and, indeed, flourish under a liberal state, though others will not. For example, ideals of the good life that are in principle open to everyone, whatever one's cultural or religious background, may well be stronger in a liberal state than are sectarian ideals that are exclusionary. Exclusionary ideals, especially when they threaten public welfare and civility, do not flourish in a liberal state, not because the liberal state cannot support their values, but because the liberal state exists for the purpose of *procedurally* restraining the sectarian forces bent on forcefully imposing particular points of view on nonadherents (Larmore 1987: 44).

This commitment involves neutrality about (nonliberal) ideals or values. It comprises a modus vivendi that requires the accommodation of difference that is characteristic of liberal societies (Larmore 1987: 74). This position is adopted to solve specific problems that arise when competing religious or political commitments threaten liberal society. It is decidedly *not* a substantive position that expresses a full ethical theory of final purposes and values. Neutrality constitutes a modus vivendi between persons whose ultimate ideals are, or could be, incompatible or fundamentally in conflict. Its very existence assumes that other substantive beliefs and values exist outside liberal theory. Autonomy understood as negative freedom is the core commitment of liberal theory. It is a profoundly political and legal commitment that regulates public interactions; it is not necessarily a defining substantive value in other sectors of everyday life. The modus vivendi view of political neutrality accepts that substantive views of what constitutes the good exist outside the political realm. This view of neutrality and the meaning of autonomy differs importantly from its opposite, the expressivist perspective.

The *expressivist perspective* understands political neutrality as the expression of a fundamental kind of detachment that humans should have if they are to flourish. The neutrality of the liberal state on this view is thus not simply a corollary to autonomy understood as negative freedom in the realm of politics, but as the highest personal ideal. On this interpretation, independence and distance from particular substantive commitments, goals, or values underpins, indeed justifies, the neutrality characteristic of the liberal state. Clearly, the expressivist defense of negative freedom must rely on a positive account of the nature of the autonomous subject. The positive model of the self that is defended by expressivists is remarkably consonant with views of the self as conceived in political theory, but it would be a mistake to attribute to political theory alone the deficiencies of the expressivist view of the self as a fundamentally detached and functioning entity. The sources of this account are much more diverse and complex. At bottom, expressivist accounts of the nature of autonomy provide a remarkably abstract and austere picture of what it means to be a self or agent in the world. Whether this abstraction is ultimately motivated by political theory, a misguided ethical theory, or other considerations is a question that need not detain us. Whatever its origin, this point of view is important for long-term care, because it affords an extremely thin and abstract account of what it is to be a person needing long-term care and of the resources that autonomy provides in constructing an ethics of long-term care. Whatever its theoretical roots, this point of view does express deep cultural attitudes in the West about the person as an agent that deserve further discussion in subsequent chapters.

There are, to be sure, other reasons to question, if not reject, the expressivist account (Larmore 1987; Young 1986). The standard criticisms of the construction of an ethics of autonomy on the basis of negative freedom are typically based on a set of wide-ranging arguments about the nature of ethics and politics. Although I draw on these wider discussions, I reference them only to the extent that they helpfully apply to the special problem of conceptualizing autonomy in the context of long-term care. The expressivist and modus vivendi perspectives provide competing views of the nature of the state in supporting particular systems of belief and value, including religious and secular systems. The modus vivendi position keeps the main themes of liberal theory intact without the (expressivist) commitment to a view of the self and the good life dependent ultimately on a view of autonomy as negative freedom. Positive accounts of autonomy are still possible, though such accounts will necessarily be ethical and not political in intent.

On this view of liberal theory, then, neutrality is a *political* ideal. Individual freedom is protected by the state procedurally by political and legal mechanisms to allow private relations to develop without constraint. For this reason, political freedom is a relatively restricted concept. It covers only the right of the person to be free of interference by the state. This negative concept has a positive component as well that is sometimes overlooked in libertarian positions: the state is not only constrained not to act, but is also obligated to assure that others (e.g., individuals or groups) also respect this right of individuals to be left alone. Hence, the negative freedom to be left alone frequently requires more than mere forbearance; it also requires the establishment of mechanisms to enforce this right. Costs are always associated with the enforcement or protection of the right to freedom. Thus, negative or liberty rights are not free, as is sometimes claimed. In an ideal world, only forbearance would be required, but practically more than forbearance has to be involved, because some individuals are by disposition or choice not willing to tolerate the beliefs or actions of others. Thus, protection of liberty entails costs that themselves involve restrictions of liberty. For example, to assure public safety and protection of rights requires the establishment of a police force, which, in turn, requires resources that are paid for by taxation. Even Isaiah Berlin's classic treatment of the concept of liberty (1969: 118–62) regarded negative liberty as a political ideal that did not exhaust everything that is reasonably included under the term *freedom*. Ronald Dworkin's critique of negative freedom is particularly pertinent (1977). Dworkin argues that there is no general right to liberty. There are only rights to specific liberties that are compatible with the equality of concern and respect for all. Liberties are thus grounded in terms of the fundamental equality of persons as bearers of rights, not in terms of a self, regarded as irremediably individual and isolated. The fundamental principle involved in Dworkin's account is thus a relational one, not just in the formal sense that equality is a principle that is applied to all persons, but substantively in that both concern and respect constitute obligatory ethical responses to other persons (Christiansen 1983: 158).

Dworkin's argument thus pairs respect with concern. Respect for persons has been interpreted by many liberal thinkers as requiring nothing more than forbearance, namely, honoring a person's negative right to noninterference. Dworkin argues that *respect* involves treating others as 'human beings who are capable of forming and acting on intelligent conceptions of how their lives should be lived' and *concern* involves treating others as 'human beings who are capable of suffering and frustration' (Dworkin 1977: 278). As a fundamental ethical attitude, concern requires that people be alert to the deprivation of others and be ready and available to relieve their deprivation whenever that is possible. In the absence of clear cases of suffering and deprivation, the principle of respect requires deference to the capacity of humans for forming and acting on intelligent conceptions of how their lives should be lived. Dworkin's analysis thus provides an important place for concern for others and the principle of equality.

Some writers have questioned the distinction between the negative and positive of liberty (Feinberg 1973; MacCallum 1967), arguing that they cannot be analyzed independently, even though the tendency of many thinkers is to do just that. In what should the positive ideals of freedom consist is certainly a matter of considerable dispute. In terms of the modus vivendi view discussed above, the state and political authorities are precluded from supporting any one candidate over all others. This statement, of course, should not be interpreted to mean that promotion of positive freedom and rights is excluded by liberal theory. Rather, liberal theory does not afford anything more than a procedural basis for addressing these questions. Instead, the issue is marked out as properly a matter of ethics, not a matter to be imposed politically. The important feature of neutrality for present purposes is that it is a uniquely *political* ideal. It governs the public relations between persons and the state or political authorities, not the private relations of persons with each other or with institutions.

Negative freedom, the freedom to pursue one's own choices without interference, is thus a uniquely political ideal. This political ideal, however, does seem to be the model for our society's understanding of individual autonomy. The autonomous state is classically characterized as independence from the laws and governance of other states. To be autonomous in this original political meaning of the term, then, is to be sovereign or to have an unfettered authority within a specific political domain or sphere of action, no matter what other conditions prevail (Young 1986: 7).

Influenced by this ideal, individual autonomy is sometimes regarded analogously as involving independence from any and all external authority including the state, institutions, or other individuals. Autonomy so regarded has obvious affinities with the concept of negative liberty articulated by Isaiah Berlin (1969: 122), namely, that to be at liberty is to be unobstructed by others. It also has affinities with those theories of rights as defining spheres of activities in which interference by others is illegitimate (Richards 1981; Wellman 1985: 102). Most versions of this political model of state autonomy, however, contain the serious deficiency of failing to account for the fact that various enabling material or empirical conditions, such as economic development, can make it impossible for states to control their own destinies in meaningful ways even though they continue to make and administer their own laws (Young 1986: 7). Thus, even at the level of the state, the model of autonomy as negative freedom is somewhat simplistic.

Economic conditions can also severely restrict the options open to individuals and so restrict their liberty in important ways (Feinberg 1978). Such restriction seems an essential and pre-given empirical fact that any fully adequate theory of autonomy needs to accommodate. Such restrictive conditions, however, are seldom given serious attention by liberal theorists who may grant passing acknowledgment that they exist even though their theories do little to incorporate these restrictions into the meaning of autonomy. There are many reasons for this omission, but they share the common feature, namely, that liberal accounts typically operate at a level of abstraction that is far removed from actual everyday reality. They tend to dwell at the level of theory, not phenomena or everyday experience. This abstract orientation creates special problems for long-term care, because the everyday detail of actual cases and circumstances of autonomy tend to get washed out in the application of the concept of autonomy. To reassess autonomy in long-term care requires that autonomy be reconceived in a way that can restore the actual features of everyday choice and action that seem to be omitted from liberal theory and incorporate into the picture of what it means to be autonomous the limitations that are concretely present in everyday life. For the moment, it is important to be clear how liberal theory typically understands the relationship of the state and positive expressions of autonomy, because these views underlie many discussions of autonomy in bioethics and, by extension, long-term care.

The distinction between the public and the private alluded to in the foregoing analysis is likely to prove troublesome for some. They might incorrectly interpret the distinction as implying that the proper ethical thrust of autonomy in long-term care rests in the private sphere. They would insist that the private sphere might generate the ethical problems associated with long-term care, but surely not their solutions. Surely, they might insist, a significant amount of institutional long-term care is public, not private. It is public in the sense that it is funded with government monies and it represents a social commitment grounded in justice of a liberal society to its elders (Daniels 1988). Analogously, they might even insist that home care is not entirely private, because public funding and regulations properly ensure that the state is nearby to scrutinize the services that are received even in the home. To insist on the prominence of the private over the public in the context of long-term care would thus be otiose. Buttressing this criticism is the insistence in the foregoing analysis that autonomy is best analyzed as an ethical and not a political/legal concept. They would rightly insist that an ethical analysis of autonomy in long-term care must have political implications. A practical treatment of autonomy in long-term care must address the concrete problems involved in meeting the health-care needs of elders. These observations are true enough, but the criticism is premature. The critics do not sufficiently note that the distinction between the public and the private is deeper and more complicated than their criticisms imply. Influenced by liberal theory, autonomy is often treated in bioethics as a concept that primarily applies to the public realm in which relationships are best described as relations with strangers as opposed to the private realm or communities (Engelhardt 1986, 1991, 1997). Individuals are thus afforded a treatment based on the minimal demands of a common and shared morality, but it is a morality that is deficient. The language of autonomy in the political/legal realm is important precisely because it finds expression in terms of various rights and corresponding obligations that prevent one community from imposing its values and beliefs on others. Such rights protect individuals by defining noninterference as a primary principle regulating interactions in the public realm. In care-giving situations, however, noninterference is a remarkably weak ethical principle that does not provide sufficient practical guidance to those inclined to or charged with the care of dependent elders. Thus, the distinction between the private and the public is one way to force the analysis away from the commonly accepted liberal view of autonomy interpreted in terms of negative freedom and noninterference and toward a more robust account of what it means ethically to respect the autonomy of an individual requiring long-term care. For the same reason, the distinction between the political and the ethical is not intended to denigrate the rule of law or political authority. Rather, it is to point out that the dominant liberal view of autonomy is primarily political and, so, an unlikely source for the ethical analysis needed in the context of long-term care.

Caregiving involves varying degrees of intimacy and affective interaction that cannot be regulated by a principle that inflexibly pits caregiver and client against one another. (I discuss this point further in the section, *Nursing Home Admission Practices.*) Hence, a concern to enhance and protect the autonomy of elders in such circumstances must turn from political and legal articulations of autonomy toward other models for guidance. Doing so, however, must confront the question of the role of the state in the promotion of positive features of autonomy.

The state and positive autonomy

The role of the state, according to liberal theory, primarily should be to enhance the ability of individuals to freely pursue their chosen life-style and preferences. Liberal theory thus strongly supports the right of elders – along with that of other competent adults – to decide what constitutes their own best interests. This theory extends even to the point of supporting the right of individuals to refuse life-sustaining treatment. For the most part, however, the freedoms defended by liberal theory are negative, namely, freedom from the interference of others. The right to refuse life-sustaining treatment is thus primarily a right not to endure the burden of advanced medical life supportive technologies. It trumps the claimed professional obligation to administer these life supportive technologies. As discussed earlier, it is commonly, though mistakenly, assumed – for example by libertarians – that the liberal state is prevented from defining positive rights or entitlements since providing such rights necessarily entails restriction on the liberty of others because of the costs associated with providing the entitlements. A minimal state that guaranteed procedural rights supporting independence, however, is not necessarily required by liberal theory, though it may first appear to be its most obvious instantiation. It is widely acknowledged that other, more enlarged roles for the state in defining positive rights are also compatible with liberal theory. Assuring fair access to a basic minimum of health care is one example in which a liberal state could legitimately structure social institutions to achieve positive outcomes (Agich 1991; Buchanan 1991; Daniels 1985, 1988; President's Commission 1983).

In the case of long-term care, the services provided might be predicated on the recognition that suffering from disabling conditions in old age represents a fundamental assault on autonomy that a liberal society should provide. The services provided, however, should be compatible with a variety of alternative normative moral beliefs and commitments. They should, in other words, be nonsectarian and should be designed to enable individuals, insofar as practically possible, to exercise independent choices or to live out their old age in terms of their unique value commitments and beliefs. Thus, a proper understanding of liberal theory would recognize that elders not only enjoy a liberty right to noninterference or correlative rights like informed consent and treatment refusal in the health care context, but also an array of social and medical systems designed to support their autonomy. Saying this is not to deny that intergenerational justice and the moral claim to resource distribution across the life span remain theoretically controversial (Agich 2001; Callahan 1985, 1987; Daniels 1988). Substantively expansive visions of the state, therefore, are not prohibited by liberal theory even though widely shared assumptions about the nature of the liberal state have historically influenced many thinkers to conclude just the opposite.

The evolution of the idea of a neutral state was influenced historically as much by beliefs that the free market was the most effective way to produce and distribute wealth and resources as by any logical requirements of liberal political theory itself. The conditions of a free market and the requirements of a liberal state became affiliated to such an extent that they are frequently identified even though nothing in liberal theory specifically requires the existence of a free market. Indeed, one might cynically point out that the rhetoric of the free market is frequently used to oppose egalitarian or redistributivist programs for the less fortunate such as welfare, but not government programs such as trade policies that help special interests. Thinking that political neutrality logically entails a free market, and by implication excludes all state involvement, shows the extent to which neutrality is seen as a substantive rather than a procedural requirement. Expressivist positions are especially prone to this mistake, which is why it is essential that we avoid these commitments.

A liberal state, especially on the modus vivendi view, is not logically precluded from actively structuring social institutions, including the market, to achieve ends justified on liberal grounds. Although individuals are free to decide what is in their best interest and what unique beliefs and values should guide their personal lives, it may be necessary for the state to provide a set of basic services in order to enable individuals to be able to pursue their vision of the good life. A liberal state can legitimately structure social institutions to achieve substantive outcomes such as assuring fair access to education, employment opportunity, housing, or health care. Health care is thus one among many such areas. In fact, the role of the state in the regulation of certain aspects of long-term care is already quite evident. Rather than considering such regulation as intrusive on theoretical grounds, it is better to ask whether the regulations in place achieve the kind of outcomes that a liberal state should support. To answer this question adequately, a positive account of the meaning of autonomy in long-term care is necessary. Before such an account can be developed, it is important to be clear why some liberal thinkers have reservations about positive accounts of autonomy.

Some problems with positive autonomy

Many liberal thinkers give primacy to negative liberty, even to the point of rejecting positive concepts of liberty as inevitably involving a totalitarian or authoritarian stance (Berlin 1969: 131). It is also sometimes said in defense of the primacy of negative liberty that positive views of autonomy necessarily entail an unjustified commitment to a metaphysical postulate regarding a real or higher self, what Isaiah Berlin termed the *inner citadel* (1969: 135–41). It is claimed that to speak of *positive* autonomy requires that one be able to differentiate a real or essential self from superficial or phenomenal expressions (Young 1986: 5). Others, however, have trenchantly argued that the liberal suspicion and criticism of positive autonomy are largely unjustified (Larmore 1987; Young 1986). Liberal theory does not logically preclude positive treatments of autonomy. The specific concerns about authoritarian and metaphysical commitments in positive accounts of autonomy, however, merit further discussion, particularly in the context of institutional long-term care, where worries about the abuse of power abound. If autonomy is to be preserved and defended in institutional long-term care, its meaning must be disentangled from these controversial implications.

The alleged authoritarian or paternalistic dangers associated with positive accounts of autonomy need to be balanced by the requirement of concern for frail elders. Simply to rely on the core liberal understanding of autonomy as negative freedom or independence without inquiring into its practical implications and significance for frail or disabled elders demonstrates a questionable apathy or insincerity at best. Such attitudes need to be set aside before the question of the ethics of long-term care can be addressed with any seriousness. Nonetheless, there is good reason to accept the (limited) relevance of traditional worries about authoritarian propensity nestled in positive accounts of autonomy and its values. For one thing, practices like the reliance on restraints to prevent injury of confused, cognitively impaired, or wandering elders need serious rebuttal (Collopy 1995; Demitrack, Lucy, and Tourigny 1988). One obvious way to do so is by attacking the authoritarian or paternalistic stance of the self-designated protectors. Correlatively, if autonomy is properly given a central place in the ethics of long-term care, it should be based on reasons that are compatible with the general commitments of liberal theory and not on some alternative foundation.

The suspicion that a suppressed metaphysical commitment regarding higher senses of self underlies positive accounts of autonomy is not a rarified philosophical or theoretical concern, but a concern that bears directly on the practical reality of long-term care. Elders requiring long-term care suffer from many kinds of disabling conditions, including severe ones like dementia. These conditions bring into question the applicability of any standard that involves reference to higher capacities. Does reference to a higher or truer self refer to an actual or ideal entity, a past or present entity or state? The attention to precedent autonomy in the bioethics literature confirms that this question has important practical implications (Blustein 1999; Buchanan 1988; Davis 2002; Kuhse 1999; Newton 1999; Quante 1999). If positive accounts of autonomy require a view of an intact self, how could they helpfully clarify cases of dementia or severe confusion? These questions are significant. Worries about paternalism and metaphysical commitments are serious enough to merit attention in any treatment of autonomy in long-term care that is broadly liberal in intent and that purports a positive vision of autonomy. Both the limitations and positive implications of the liberal model of autonomy for long-term care thus require further exploration.

Liberal principles in long-term care

Liberal thought expresses fundamental cultural attitudes regarding not only liberty but also what it ultimately means to be a person, which cannot be lightly dismissed. The liberal defense of autonomy as negative freedom has its proper place in the restricted realms of politics and law, leaving to ethics the task of providing a positive account of autonomy. This strategy was admirably defended in Charles Larmore's (1987) argument that liberal theory is primarily a political not an ethical theory. When properly confined to politics and law, liberal principles are both plausible and defensible. Their unbridled extension into the realm of ethics, however, leads to unsatisfactory, even repugnant, outcomes. The challenge for a positive account of autonomy in long-term care is to develop an ethical framework that supplements, rather than rejects, the liberal view. It should support liberal concerns by offering a fuller account of what autonomy involves in the world of everyday life. Because the view of patient autonomy and rights that is commonplace in bioethics is primarily liberal in nature, our analysis of autonomy in long-term care must be careful not to reintroduce the limitations of liberal theory through this back door. Instead, we need to ask whether the concept of autonomy has relevance for long-term care independent of the taken-for-granted commitments common in mainstream bioethics and, more importantly, to develop a framework for thinking about autonomy that provides practical guidance for the long-term care.

Despite the limitations and complications just discussed, liberal ideas about autonomy are salient in long-term care. The liberal version of autonomy provides a historically important foundation for the establishment of certain rights to information, privacy, and so on that are as important in long-term care as in other contexts of health care and social life. Such rights globally serve to assure that elders are not forced to adopt values or visions of the good life that are not their own. In their most general form, these rights are the (negative) right to noninterference. In ethical terms, such a right reminds us that nonmaleficence is more basic in many contexts as a principle of action than beneficence. Not affecting individuals in ways that they would judge harmful is more important than pursuing a particular good for individuals if the persons in question would refuse to acknowledge or accept the outcome as good. Although these points are widely accepted, their application in long-term care is not straightforward.

A strong reading of liberal principles seems to imply that individuals have what has been termed in the psychiatric context a *right to rot* (Appelbaum and Gutheil 1979; Gutheil and Appelbaum 1980). When the liberty principle is taken as fundamental, then the right to be left alone is maximized without regard for the actual condition of the individual and without regard for the harm that results. Such a right would support the abandonment of elders to their illnesses, disabilities, and distress. It would provide a general basis for ignoring the plight of helpless individuals. This would lead one, paradoxically, to insist on the right of elders to be left alone in the name of autonomy, when interventions, such as providing transportation, could actually expand the range of action and choice of elders. Such an outcome is highly undesirable and, indeed, ethically repugnant. For this reason, many have tried to argue against liberalism and the liberal ideals of pluralism and toleration by insisting that communitarian considerations relocate individual choice within its proper social context (Gauthier 2000; Kegley 1999). Insisting on the importance of the value and principle of care or relationship, some thinkers have sought to correct problems with autonomy (Donchin 2000; Parks 1998; Sailors 2001). These moves risk throwing out the baby with the bath water, since the real problem is the unbridled scope accorded the specific principle of negative freedom, not the broad liberal view in which neutrality and toleration are understood to be foundational political principles. In this regard, recent work considers whether tolerance rather than autonomy is a more reliable foundation for liberal political theory (Gilbert 2000).

The liberal view of autonomy does provide a broad political and legal framework by which the state ensures that dependent individuals should not be subject to discrimination and that they should be protected from the unwanted intrusions of others. That implication is generally defensible. The liberal view of autonomy provides the theoretical foundation for the principles of informed consent and respect for patients that are salutary developments in medical ethics. Generally, the creation and implementation of patient rights are positive outcomes that are admirably defended by the liberal principle of autonomy, though it should be acknowledged that confining discussion to such rights does raise a host of dilemmas such as the problem of determining competence (Macklin 1983a, 1983b), weaknesses that many standard accounts of autonomy usually finesse. Two examples readily illustrate the relevance of autonomy as negative freedom to long-term care: nursing home admission practices and the use of physical and other restraints.

Nursing home admission practices

Whatever the reasons, nursing home admissions are characteristically stressful; they often occur in circumstances of crisis. No matter what reasons justify the admission, it is frequently final because of transfer trauma and inertia (Taylor 1981). Admission of an elder to a nursing home is often a one-way passage. In many circumstances, the elders' choice of residence is limited by the availability of a nursing home bed and by the willingness of many nursing homes to accept patients unable to pay full charges. Typically, elders themselves are seldom actively involved in the admissions process. Elders typically are admitted; they do not admit themselves. Even when clearly competent, elders are frequently not asked to sign their own admission contract (Ambrogi and Gerard 1986; Buckingham 1987). Investigation of nursing home admission contracts has concluded that they typically contain unlawfully restrictive language and that elders and their representatives are rarely fully aware of their content or the implications of the agreement that they sign (Ambrogi 1990; Ambrogi and Gerard 1986; Ambrogi and Leonard 1988a, 1988b; Legal Services for the Elderly 1983; Schneider and Oliver 1987; Subcommittee on Law and the Elderly 1987). Virtually all nursing home admission agreements are adhesion contracts, standardized form contracts that are characterized by unequal power relations (Ambrogi 1990: 73). Although theoretically subject to negotiation, these contracts are usually offered on a take-it or leave-it basis. Many contracts misrepresent the extent of the institution's liability under the law and do not specifically list what services elders and their families can expect to be provided. The contracts contain exculpatory clauses or waivers that seek to limit liability or excuse the institution altogether for the negligence of its staff or attending physicians, for injury caused to a resident by another resident or by wandering away from the institution, for theft of personal property, or damage to personal property caused by smoking. The effect of this misrepresentation is to intimidate and discourage elders from pursuing valid claims (Brown 1985; Nemore 1985). Although such waiver clauses are not legally enforceable, they may be practically effective in shielding the facility from lawsuit. Ambrogi points out that most contracts omit definitions of key terms such as the services specifically included in the daily rate; as a result, the monthly charge incurred can exceed what is claimed to be the basic daily rate.

Some agreements even contain clauses that conflict with the Bill of Rights. The most common clause requires residents to agree in advance to a broad range of medical treatment and diagnostic procedures (Ambrogi and Gerard 1986). These blanket consents allegedly empower the institution's staff to diagnose or treat conditions on the basis of their professional discretion without the need for any further decision by the elder or the elder's surrogate decision maker. Some contracts are required to be signed by a so-called responsible party or guarantor, who assumes not only a personal financial liability for the elder as a requirement of admission, but also medical decision-making authority. Such practices seem to violate statutory procedures regarding surrogate health care decision making in many states and fundamentally abridge the right of elders to fully informed consent. A financial guarantor may not be the legal guardian of the patient, yet the financial guarantor's signature on an admission agreement is taken to constitute appropriate consent for admission. Ambrogi reports that other rights are regularly infringed in admission agreements; these rights include confidentiality of medical records, elders' right of access to records, the right to patronize a pharmacy of one's choice, the right to receive visitors of all ages at reasonable times, the right to privacy with respect to photographs, the right to reasonable policies regarding smoking and personal furnishings, and the right of access to nonfacility food and drink (1990: 74).

In analyzing these abuses, the language of rights is undeniably significant. To have a right to something, however, does not mean that it is morally good to pursue that object or to enjoy its possession. It is important that the distinction between possessing a right and the morally justified exercise of a right should not be overlooked. For example, although an elder has a right to refuse institutionalization in order to protect her sense of negative freedom, to do so in the face of family concern and her inability to care for herself in any minimally adequate matter requires justification beyond the simple appeal to the individual's right to refuse institutionalization. The right to be left alone establishes what is *morally permitted*; it does not establish that its own exercise is *morally justified* in the circumstances. Insisting on basic rights in the admissions process and the protection of legal rights during institutionalization should not obscure the fact that the defensible exercise of rights, whatever the right might be, is itself an ethically valid question. While the violation of the legal rights of elders in the process of admission is indefensible, pointing out and correcting these deficiencies by appealing to the concept of liberty do not provide an ethically sound framework from which to approach the complex issues associated with nursing home admission.

The use of restraints

The presence of questionable admission practices nevertheless reinforces the lure of negative freedom and emphasizes the positive role that the values of self-determination and noninterference that are basic to our legal system and medical ethics can have on nursing home care. In a similar fashion, the use of physical restraints infringes on an obvious sense of autonomy as independence that liberals want to defend. Physical restraints are reported to be in wide use in nursing homes. These include restraining geri-chairs, waist and Posey restraints that tie the resident to a chair, as well as wrist restraints that are applied to residents at night, and side rails that prevent residents from getting out of bed (Evans and Strumpf 1989). One argument frequently used to support the use of physical restraint involves the alleged institutional liability for injury. Some negligence cases are filed alleging the failure to prevent an institutionalized elder from falling or failure to use side rails (Kapp 1987). There is little evidence that institutions have been held liable for injury simply because they failed to employ physical restraint (Kapp 1985).

Andrew Jameton (1990) pointed out that there is a strong ethical presumption against using restraints. The presumption is not based on a very sophisticated understanding of freedom of action, but involves what he termed *elemental liberty.* The activities restricted by physical restraints are so basic, he argues, that it is not easy to distinguish the ability to engage in the activities and the ability to make choices about engaging in them. The capacity for action is often regarded as more a matter of physical competence and the decision or choice is a mental competence. In activities like walking, and sitting, and standing, the two competencies merge. To be physically restrained is to be rendered physically unable to act and so unable to make a meaningful choice regarding action (Jameton 1990: 167). On this view, then, there is a basic presumption against the use of restraints that derives from the most basic understanding of autonomy as negative freedom.

Restraints also increase a person's vulnerability to harm, exploitation, and neglect. They restrict physical motion and so the ability of elders to protect themselves. In some instances, they constitute a danger to the elder. Perhaps more importantly, physical restraint is not the only way to deal with the problem. Changing the structure of the environment (Cohen and Weisman 1990) can also obviate problems that are sometimes wrongly attributed to the elder. For example, one might lower a bed if the protective rails make the elder anxious (Blakeslee, Goldman, and Papougenis 1990).

Jameton pointed out that a crucial element in the ethics of the use of restraints involves the degree of voluntariness involved. Seat belts provide a good contrast to restraints. Not only does their use serve life and health, they also serve the choice of safety over risk. In the case of nursing home use of restraints, however, it is often difficult to identify the degree of voluntariness involved. The background circumstances of involuntary admission, physical and mental impairment, and the profound control by nursing home staff of the rules and activities of daily life make the question of willingness to be restrained difficult to assess. Appeal to the liberal principle of noninterference helps to establish the basic ethical presumption against the use of restraints in the first place. The complication is that this presumption can be overridden. Good reasons exist for using restraints in some circumstances, for example for protection of the elder from serious harm. The initial appeal of negative freedom is thus considerably diminished. The ethically interesting, and indeed perplexing, questions arise if we are willing to look beyond this basic presumption. Jameton (1990) argued that six factors are ethically relevant in making decisions to restrain elders: the frequency and intensity of danger posed to others, the frequency and intensity of danger posed to self, the wishes of the elder, the mental competence of the elder, the comfort of the elder with the restraints, and the wishes of the family. Considering these factors forces us to step beyond the concept of negative autonomy and toward the more positive concept of what it means to be a person who is vulnerable with responsibilities to self and others. The typical strong appeal to negative freedom can stymie the construction of a positive framework of autonomy.

Simply prohibiting the use of restraints without further analysis and discussion is not ethically sufficient, because restraints can be a justified response to genuine problems in the care of some elders. Assuring safety and preventing injury must be accounted for in any adequate analysis of the problematic use of restraints. Beyond the concept of protection, a positive framework for understanding autonomy would address in this context the meaning of wandering in the life of the elder before the risk of injury associated with falls can be properly assessed. The application of an expansive liberal understanding of autonomy can usurp other considerations that are ethically relevant in considering the problem of restraints.

The perils of liberal theory

One significant deficiency with the standard liberal view of autonomy for long-term care is that it supports an abstract view of persons as independent, self-sufficient centers of decision making. In a sense, such individuals become absolute centers of decision making. One consequence is that individuals express or are seen to express preferences and decisions that they take to be absolutely binding in all relationships (Toulmin 1981). No wonder, then, that disagreements often engender conflicts and disputes that cannot be settled by appeal to further principles, shared belief, or rational discourse and negotiation. Autonomy thus becomes more an obsession than a moral principle (Callahan 1984).

This cultural fixation on autonomy is directly evident in the prominence given to patient rights in bioethics. Patient rights constrain medical intervention unless explicit consent is given. In compromised and debilitated elders, especially those who are confused or demented, explicit consent may be an unattainable ideal. Since the requirement of consent derives from the principle of autonomy, it is often treated as ethically beyond question, though it is easy to see that this is wrong. Steven H. Miles described the case of his 94-year-old great aunt who refused cataract surgery despite assurances that it was a minor, outpatient procedure (Miles 1988). Her refusal was related to her belief that if she went to the hospital she would die, as did her mother 50 years earlier from a septic gallbladder. Miles, a physician, felt torn between respecting his aunt's autonomy (and her right to be free from the interference of strangers) on the one hand and his sense of responsibility and desire to help as a nephew on the other. As Miles expressed it:

as an absolute, autonomy reveals an impoverished view of how we live and are sustained in moral communities. On balance, the 'autonomy ethic' serves many persons well. But, the epitaph of 'It's their responsibility' is a facile way to blame those not served by this standard and excuse us from their need for our care. (1988: 2583)

Although this example is, strictly speaking, an instance of an acute care decision, it should not be forgotten that such crises are common in long-term care. In such situations, the family or guardian is asked to make decisions on behalf of the elder. Leaving aside the question of whether the elder is presently competent or not, one can ask, 'Does autonomy afford any substantive moral guidance for such decisions?' On the model of autonomy as negative freedom, the answer is clearly no. Even when the patient is competent, as in Miles's case, autonomy affords a justification that is only satisfactory in the abstract. In fact, what is at the heart of Miles's case is the morally destitute position created by the sheer lack of fundamental concern or sympathy for the other that standard understandings of the meaning of autonomy seem to offer. If autonomy is to be a relevant consideration in such cases, a positive account will be necessary to provide an ethically substantive basis for decision making.

Analogous problems occur in the everyday world of long-term care (Kane and Caplan 1990). Although the consequences of honoring a putatively autonomous choice of or simply providing care are less dramatic, they are nonetheless ethically significant. For example, how is autonomy relevant to deciding what degree and kinds of protections, including restraints, are appropriate for elders who are confused, cognitively impaired, or demented? Is it more important to afford institutionalized elders choices, for example from a range of routine in-house social activities, such as bingo, crafts, or the once-a-month communal birthday party, or is it more important that the options available be meaningful for the particular elders involved? Playing bingo may be one of the few regular group activities available for nonambulatory elders. If bingo (or other organized social activities) is seen by a particular elder as meaningless or even offensive, then the very act of affording the choice, including the opportunity to consider the option and freely decide whether or not to participate, could diminish, even though subtly, the elder's sense of self-worth and magnify the alienation. Although such an outcome is regrettable, is it a problem of autonomy?

When an elder prefers to sit in a nearby park where good weather might be enjoyed or where watching birds, squirrels, or children can be enjoyed, but the nursing home does not afford safe access, then is the existence of a choice between bingo or some activity occurring within the nursing home an adequate respect of the elder's autonomy? If the elder in question suffers from confusional states, is a trip to the park, no matter how much an elder insists on it, a defensible option that should be honored just because it is the free choice of the elder? Are there other factors to consider besides the mere fact of choice or preference in respecting autonomy? Responses that simply insist on autonomy as the free exercise of choice in these examples to the exclusion of other factors are ethically unsatisfactory, though as yet it is not evident why this is true; or, if it is true, what it has to do with autonomy.

Implied in the foregoing is the view that if autonomy as negative freedom is not restricted to the political/legal realm, but is permitted to dominate the ethical analysis of long-term care, then the practical ethical problems associated with long-term care will be oversimplified. The rich terrain of the everyday world of long-term care will be flattened and made more monotonous than it now appears. Even if we pursue the ideal of autonomy as negative freedom for elders by various procedural devices like nursing home preadmission agreements, the deeper ethical questions of autonomy in long-term care and its apparent loss or alteration in dependent states are left to one side. Addressing these questions, however, seems an essential requirement for any treatment of autonomy that purports to adequately reflect the reality of long-term care.

The concept of negative freedom is like a herd of cattle when allowed to roam outside its normal range; it inevitably tramples without discrimination both the flowers and weeds of everyday ethical life. The widespread cultural belief that independence and noninterference exhaust all that can be meaningfully said about autonomy should not be accepted. Some critics of the likened theory of autonomy say that the idolatry of the individual is at the root of this problem, but such idolatry may be more the symptom than the cause. One intellectually serious elaboration of this attitude has involved the search for an alternative ethic, one that decisively rejects the liberal value of autonomy as independence. Much of this effort has been conducted under the emblem of communitarianism.

Communitarianism and the contextualist alternative

Communitarianism is a motley movement that broadly involves a critique of liberal individualism and autonomy, as well as the permissiveness that it promotes and appeals to ideas and ideals of community, tradition, and virtue as foundational elements in ethics (Bellah et al. 1985; Hauerwas 1981; MacIntyre 1981, 1988; Perry 1988; Sandel 1982). Communitarians typically argue that autonomy is not a definitive or fundamental value nor is it universally accepted; it is a product of a certain historical epoch, the Enlightenment or Age of Modernity. For this reason, among many, they claim that the alleged universal and nonsectarian quality attributed to autonomy by liberal theorists is largely a matter of historical amnesia. Communitarians typically argue for a view of ethics that focuses on the formation of character rather than on the possession of rights and obligations. Ethics thus is defined primarily in terms of virtues that are understood in terms of a teleological unity of life that is anchored in the concept of a tradition.

Individual selves are not independent centers of decision making, but are the product of history that is communal. The individual self is thus essentially bound up with membership in communities, such as those of family, neighborhood, city, tribe, or nation. That means that the self finds its moral identity in and through membership in these various communities. In a sense, then, individuals are never unformed or independent, but exist primarily through identifications with others. The actions and choices of individuals reflect the values of their community. For this to occur, communitarians assume that a tradition involves a high degree of moral consensus not just about particular beliefs and values, but about the final purposes and nature of human life (MacIntyre 1988). Individuals fit within this all encompassing structure just as episodes in a story fit within the larger narrative structure. Hence, individual human lives have unity, purpose, and meaning insofar as they exhibit a kind of narrative structure that links them to traditional values rather than being independent centers of choice.

Individuals are understood in terms of the kind of lives they live comparable with the kind of stories their lives tell about them. Communitarians think that the kind of stories open to individuals to exhibit in their lives is limited by the given community's particular and determinate beliefs about the ultimate purpose of human life. These beliefs define the shared tradition that gives form and purpose to individual existence. Drawing on these purposes and values, individuals are sustained in their everyday existence. The final purpose and nature of human life are seen as essentially articulated in tradition that is the foundational repository of authority for making moral judgments. In other words, tradition provides a privileged and not a relative access to transcendent truths and values needed for ethics.

An implication of communitarian thought is that individualism and autonomy are deficient ideals, because they sever individuals from the cultural and historical tradition that persons need to sustain themselves as moral agents. Communitarians often insist that instead of free choice and independence, acceptance of the authority of tradition or authorities within the community should be encouraged. Persons are said to realize their true nature and purpose only insofar as they exhibit the traits and virtues that allow them to participate in the wider reality of tradition and community. To be a moral agent is thus to place oneself in the bosom of the larger community, because only the community can provide the ultimate moral meaning of human life and action. An important implication of these views is that the transcendent reality of human nature is available as a source and guide for the ethical life of individuals only as it is authoritatively interpreted by the community (Hauerwas 1982; Veatch 1982).

Despite its strengths, communitarianism exhibits one seriously deficient philosophical assumption that renders it a nonviable option, namely, its view that a contextual justification of ethical belief or action cannot be established objectively (Larmore 1987: 27–35). Communitarians regularly assume that the objectivity of a particular moral belief can be established only if the whole of our moral beliefs can be justified, only if we can show that *as a whole* they justify or make sense of human action by reference to an extramoral telos. That is why communitarian thought so readily embraces religion. This belief is, in effect, an epistemological foundationalism carried over to the realm of morality (Larmore 1987: 29). The requirement that any belief is justified only if the belief as a whole is justified is a tremendously difficult requirement for any theory to meet. Hence, it is no surprise that communitarianism cannot satisfy this requirement. No communitarian account has really succeeded in establishing the objectivity that the theory requires. Given the diversity of knowledge and traditions to which communitarians appeal, such an outcome is inevitable, though it is not adequately acknowledged by these thinkers. Unless one accepts force and rejects reason, as Engelhardt (1991) has argued, this view is unsustainable.

The concept of tradition is appealed to, but the concept of tradition is more an abstraction than a concrete, actual historical entity. Actual traditions are seldom wholly rational systems. In fact, there are good reasons to doubt whether claims about tradition *simpliciter* have anything more than rhetorical or argumentative significance in communitarian thought. According to communitarians, tradition is something within which one lives; it is not something that one puts on for the occasion like a suit of clothes; yet, it is conveniently overlooked that real traditions frequently include dissent. If dissent is to be forestalled for fear that it lead to anarchy, then appeal to tradition comes down to an appeal to some authority to settle matters of contemporary debate. Indeed, the authority appealed to must be powerful enough to impose orthodoxy and foreclose further discussion and debate.

Such a line of argument is questionable, because it displays a circularity of reasoning. It will not do simply to insist that a holistic vision or metaphysical view of the final ends or purposes of humanity is required, because that is precisely what is in dispute between communitarians and liberals. Tradition regarded abstractly is used by communitarians to bludgeon the liberal alternative into submission, while all too frequently it is overlooked that liberalism, too, can be regarded as a tradition (MacIntyre 1988).

The view that an authoritative foundation is necessary, and that such a foundation ultimately must be metaphysical or substantive, seems a common prerequisite of communitarian accounts. Although this kind of commitment is shared with expressivist brands of liberalism, the modus vivendi, contextualist, or pragmatic versions of liberal thought seem comfortable with the absence of such substantive anchors. That is not to say that these views endorse relativism, but they do acknowledge that the modern sense of foundation articulated in the work of Descartes is but one side of modem thought (Toulmin 1990). Indeed, the need felt for a foundation or anchor expresses a certain insecurity that is characteristic of modem thinking, though it is not at all clear why absolute foundations or first principles are needed to philosophically articulate a coherent world view. The debate over foundationalism is a debate about the metaphor of a foundation or anchor. The dominant metaphor is that of a land-based anchor or foundation for a building, but there are other kinds of anchor. For example, sailors in waters too deep for bottom anchors use a sea anchor. A sea anchor is a large parachute-like device that is submerged to catch the current. Such anchors steady the ship against the force of wind and waves. Flexible anchors may be the only kind of foundation that humans need achieve.

One serious criticism of liberalism made by communitarians is that the liberal view of autonomy commits one to relativism or subjectivism such that objectivity of moral belief becomes impossible to secure. In the practical context, this amounts to the claim that the only ethics possible is therefore a situational ethics, implying an objectionable relativism of value and belief. The only way to avoid such relativism, communitarians insist, is to adhere to the authority of tradition and community. Communitarianism typically rejects the view that ethics is truly a distinct realm; it rejects the idea that we attain our real humanity only in and through ethical life. Instead, communitarians often want to reestablish particular religious or theological views, for example the view that morality is the route to salvation. Hence, ethics is made dependent on religion. These approaches are properly criticized on liberal grounds as being at least potentially coercive or oppressive (Engelhardt 1991). Tyranny, not community, is often the result of such imposed religious visions of the good life, as history repeatedly demonstrates.

Both the liberal defense of the primacy of negative freedom in the sphere of ethics and the communitarian insistence on the primacy of tradition and community over individuals exhibit a common defect. Embracing tradition and community as ultimate sources of authority seems to commit the same kind of mistake that communitarians attribute to liberal thought, namely, of insisting on absolute authority; the difference is that communitarians do so on the side of the community rather than the individual. Both of these extreme views need to be rejected. The alternative to both absolutistic liberal and communitarian thought is *contextualism*, namely, the view that actions and beliefs can be justified in a rationally defensible way without having to appeal to absolute principles or theories.

Contextualism is the view that morality is properly concerned with the life of human beings who exist as finite, social creatures engaged in particular existential settings and projects. This means that justification itself is seen as a human endeavor and one that is irremediably local. There is no absolute, privileged, or completely objective standpoint from which to settle ethical disputes conclusively. The contextualist view is differentiated from both the liberal insistence on the primacy of negative freedom (and its corollary view that the individual is the final arbiter in ethics) as well as from the communitarian faith in the final authority of tradition and community.

Contextualism is not new. Aristotle, too, had argued that there are no essences in the realm of ethics. There could therefore be no basis for any scientifically rigorous or objective theory of ethics and no basis for any absolute principles of ethics. Practical reasoning in ethics, as in other practical contexts like clinical medicine, is essentially a matter of judgment. The exercise of judgment involves weighing and considering different alternatives. It is never simply a matter of formally deducing conclusions from strict or self-evident axioms or rules. Communitarian and many forms of liberal theory provide inadequate guidance to understanding autonomy in long-term care, because they essentially involve commitments to abstract views of autonomy and value.

Practical implications of the debate over the foundation of ethics

The debate over the nature of autonomy and its relation to morality is not only theoretically interesting and important, but also has practical implications for long-term care. As argued above, the liberal view of autonomy and its corollary articulation in legal rights is compatible with the criticism of that view when liberal theory is extended beyond its proper political bounds. It is thus possible to retain positive features of the liberal view of autonomy and the legal protections afforded elderly individuals, while still criticizing these views for usurping the proper concerns of ethics in long-term care. One does not need to accept communitarian thought uncritically, particularly insofar as it tends to underestimate the significance of the liberal value of protecting the rights of individuals in the public or political/legal sphere and tends to be committed to a naive foundationalism. Instead, one can look to an account of autonomy that captures some of the central tendencies and insights of communitarian thought without a monistic vision of the good life. Such an account can regard humans as social creatures who must be understood in terms of their concrete relations with one another without making tradition and community into absolute sources of moral insight and guidance.

The practical implication of this point is that the fabric of rights secured by a liberal concept of autonomy remains intact. The application of rights becomes a matter of ethical judgment and discretion. In the context of long-term care, the function of autonomy that remains vital is to provide procedural protections to assure that a range of alternative expressions of the best way to grow old, handle disability, or live out the last days of one's life is possible. This pluralistic outcome does imply, as communitarians often (though wrongly) insist, that an absolute or objective foundation necessary for ethics or the moral life is eliminated. The belief in an absolutistic foundationalist ethics must be abandoned, but a contextual ethics, the only kind ultimately possible for finite beings, is retained. This will not satisfy communitarians, but it can accommodate the central substantive contributions of communitarian thought to contemporary ethics. The crucial insight of communitarianism, namely, that the moral life is essentially social and that persons are not atomistic, self-centered, rational decision makers, but selves formed by a living tradition and culture, is unequi-vocally retained. Moral agents by definition exhibit more than independent freedom of action or choice; they manifest character and virtues. Commu-nitarians are correct because the expansive version of autonomy as negative freedom is self-defeating generally and certainly unhelpful and unworkable in the context of long-term care. Fortunately, nothing in liberal theory, properly interpreted, logically requires such an extreme conclusion anyway.

The proper interpretation of the liberal theory of autonomy is a contextualist view of liberalism that restricts negative freedom to the political/legal realm. Positive concepts of autonomy are not only possible but also necessary for ethics, but these concepts must be neutral. An account of the nature of ethical experience that is compatible with a restricted liberal theory is thus possible. Such an account is also compatible with the broad outlines of communitarian views that persons are historical and social beings and that character and virtue are important concepts in ethics. These insights prevent ethics from becoming the abstract play of principles that have the sole purpose of regulat-ing interactions among strangers (Toulmin 1981). The incursion of such an ethics of strangers into health care has had the effect of reinterpreting caring, intimacy, and other emotional attachments as prima facie evidence of objec-tionably paternalistic behavior (Cluff and Binstock 2001). It would be most unfortunate if an ethics of long-term care were to repeat these mistakes.

Respect for autonomy as independence is important in those settings in which the language of rights and principles of equity and equality are properly central. Accepting this point, however, does not make the liberal principle of autonomy and rights the cornerstone of ethics in other situations that involve intimacy or concrete and genuine moral conflict, complexity, and tragedy. If the primary function of the principle of autonomy was to make sense of and justify an adversarial legal system designed to address conflictual interactions between strangers, what would happen in situations in which the psychological outcomes were the most damaging and serious, such as in situations of conflict involving the care of children or elders? Stephen Toulmin (1981) pointed out that in areas like family law, some nations have chosen to handle disputes through arbitration rather than through litigation, in chambers rather than in open court, in order to provide as much room as possible for discretion. The focus on arbitration rather than litigation and on judgmental discretion rather than rigorism in the application of principles is especially significant, because it rightly indicates that the ethics of relationships with intimates, such as family member or acquaintances, is fundamentally different from moral relationships with complete strangers. If so, important implications follow for the ethics of long-term care in which intimacy is an important feature.

Long-term care is poorly understood if it is restricted to the ethics of re-lationships between strangers. Certainly, such relations are unavoidable in some long-term care situations. In most long-term care, however, even when strangers enter these relationships, degrees of intimacy and familiarity develop as the inevitable outcomes of continuous interaction. Indeed, when they fail to develop, something may be amiss in the social environment of caregiving. Hence, it is critically important to assess what respect for autonomy can mean in circumstances that deviate significantly from the model assumed by the dominant view of autonomy as negative freedom or independence.

One way to develop these points preliminarily is to consider how the view of autonomy as independence (and the view of inviolate patient rights that derives therefrom) is related to assumptions about the nature of medicine and health care that are further discussed in Chapter 3. Autonomy conceived in terms of independence and noninterference is recommended by certain acute care situations. These situations paradigmatically support the extension of the political/legal view of autonomy into medical ethics, but their limitation has not been fully appreciated. In much of medical ethics, the standard or paradigm cases and problems involve dramatic conflictual four-alarm cases (McCullough and Wear 1985: 296–97). Conflict and disagreement predominate and patients (as well as families) seem to be pawns in the hands of a powerful and impersonal system of medical care. It is at least arguable that long-term care involves and requires a different paradigm or framework (Agich 1990c). Such dramatic cases of conflict are less evident in long-term care. Exclusive attention to such cases diverts attention from more pervasive, interstitial aspects of everyday life that deserve to be the focus of attention (Agich 1995a; Kane and Caplan 1990).

Conflict and conversation

Preliminary to developing an alternative framework for assessing autonomy in long-term care, it is important to appreciate how certain commitments of the liberal view of autonomy also support the view that individuals are best understood in social terms, rather than as atomistic, rational decision makers. It is important to make clear that the liberal view is badly represented by the libertarian, individualistic extreme; the properly interpreted liberal view of autonomy sees individuals as historical, social beings consistent with the central focus of communitarian thought. One way to establish this point is to consider the logical requirements of neutrality and toleration in liberal theory. As Larmore put it:

Neutrality is simply a means of accommodation. It is a stance that we adopt in order to solve a specific problem to which our various commitments give rise, and so it is not a stance that expresses our full understanding of our purposes. It establishes a modus vivendi between persons whose ultimate ideals do not coincide. (1987: 74)

Several considerations recommend such a stance.

First, the norm of rational conversation requires that if we want to solve a problem but encounter disagreement about how to do so, we should retreat to neutral ground. Second, besides a desire for civil peace and sympathy for those whose ideals are similar to ours, the norm of equal respect demands that we explain our proposals to those whom they will affect, even if we believe that they will disagree. Third, our own pursuit of a substantial ideal of the good life, it seems reasonable to believe, will be protected if others, with different ideals, also agree that common political principles should be decided from neutral ground. Importantly, none of these reasons calls for any weakening of our allegiance to our personal beliefs and values or our own vision of the good life. All that is required is that we give up the conviction that our beliefs and values have ultimate validity.

When confronted by irresolvable disagreement, individuals who wish to resolve disagreements must retreat to a neutral ground with the hope of either resolving the dispute or bypassing it. This retreat to a neutral ground allows one to remain as convinced of the truth of one's views as before, but for the purposes of carrying on the conversation, one sets aside the absolute claim of these beliefs. In other words, the ideal or goal of keeping the conversation going, which is motivated by the desire to achieve some reasoned agreement about how to solve the problem at hand, gives substantive force to the ideal of neutrality (Larmore 1987: 53). For this to occur, at least two criteria must be met: first, the conditions necessary for conversation, namely, the prerequisites of communicative interaction, must be available, and, second, the desire or commitment to solve the problem at hand through reasoned agreement must override the tendency to use force to end the impasse. These conditions posit a view of individuals as historical, social beings that must, by their very nature, live together and interact.

Reason, rather than force, is compelling not because it is more effective, all things considered, but because it preserves the very conditions of interaction that each of us requires, whereas force destroys the social fabric necessary for human beings to be truly human. Although one may win a dispute by force, for example by killing one's opponent, such a maneuver makes impossible the conditions that sustain human beings in historical and social relationships. One need only consider the problems that exist around the world where people cannot overcome their differences. History repeatedly shows that force engenders rather than resolves discord in the end. Similarly, one need only look to the sorry state of many long-term care settings that rely on staff authority and power to manage their charges for ready examples of the objectionable consequences of this view. It is worth noting that even if reliance on coercion and force does not make human social existence impossible, it does reduce the qualitative possibilities, a consequence that is of equal ethical importance.

The function of rights

Appeals to autonomy often are made in situations of conflict in long-term care, such as over decisions to institutionalize, to increase levels of skilled care, or to begin, withhold, or withdraw life-prolonging medical technologies. Such appeals undoubtedly serve the important function in these contexts of curbing the pretensions and power of health care providers. The language of rights is prominent in this process of appeal: for example, the right to refuse treatment, the right to informed consent, or the right of self-determination. Rights do offer protection to individuals from the impersonal decision making of health care institutions and health professionals who hold a disproportionate share of power. A claim to rights is thus often a strong moral counterweight to a line of decision making that rests on, for example, what the rules of an institution require, what is customary in the profession or institution, or what the practitioner usually does in such cases (Agich 1982). This counterweight is undoubtedly important, but it comes into play and is significant primarily when controversy ensues or conflict arises. The language of rights thus does not tell how to avoid these circumstances, nor does it seem able to satisfactorily settle true cases of ethical conflict or dilemma. Examples of true ethical dilemmas involve fundamental conflicts of principle or value. Such cases are not settled simply by insisting on one principle over and against its competitor. Rights language implies that ethical obligations are satisfied whenever rights are honored. This implication is supported by three important logical properties that characterize rights.

First, rights claims are unique moral claims in that they are peremptory: they are absolute and bar further debate or discussion; they cannot be changed, delayed, or denied. When a person's rights are involved, many sorts of action are authorized that would otherwise be impermissible (Ladd 1978: 16). For example, it is wrong to harm another person, yet if Mr Jones tries to take my wallet, I am justified in physically preventing him from doing so even if my actions cause him injury. Even though it is morally wrong to kill, my own right to life justifies my effort to defend myself even to the extent of causing my assailant mortal harm. Second, because rights are appealed to when the person against whom the right is asserted threatens, neglects, or otherwise appears unwilling to accede to one's requests, needs, or demands, they assume that an adversarial relationship exists between the parties involved (Ladd 1978: 17; Wellman 1985: 102). Third, it is important to note that an individual possesses a right if he can choose not to exercise it. In this sense, rights are a reflection of the concept of a person as free and capable of making decisions. Decision-making capacity is simply presumed. More important for present purposes, it is also presumed that the choices available to the rights possessor are in some broad sense desirable or even sensible. That, of course, need not be the case. It is a mistake to think that the choices afforded by a right are ethically unproblematic just so long as they are afforded by a valid right. Everyday experience is rife with examples in which this does not seem to be the case. A simple example can illustrate this point.

I have a meal ticket to a cafeteria that affords an extensive menu for lunch. One day each of the main courses, desserts, and soups contains milk or milk products to which I am allergic. My right to choose is unfettered, but my actual choice is burdened with the consequences of a known food allergy; alternatively, my choice might be constrained by religion-based dietary restrictions or simply by my preferences. In either of these situations, I have a right to choose guaranteed by my legitimate possession of a meal ticket even though each of the choices available is problematic for me. Rights advocates might be quick to point out, however, that this is not much of an objection since I retain other rights that give me other options, including the liberty right to forego using my meal ticket. This is undoubtedly true, but the important point is that the attention to rights tends to adjust the focus of analysis in such a way that the concrete detail is lost, namely, that the cafeteria's offerings are inadequate or insensitive to the dietary needs of at least one of its patrons. The language of rights is largely irrelevant to what is problematic in the actual circumstances, that is, my inability to eat in the cafeteria despite my possession of a meal ticket.

Rights are typically seen as important, because of their tie to autonomy understood in terms of independence and noninterference. That is, rights are designed to afford individuals protection from the intrusion of others. The assumption seems to be that individuals need such protection because individuals as persons are best understood on their own or in their own terms, and that ethics is best understood as the effort to protect the freedom of choice. In effect, persons are construed as social and moral atoms in this view. They are represented without significant reference to their own developmental history, personal values, or relationships with others. Human relationships are thereby taken to be a secondary aspect of being a person for purposes of the theory. Relationships are considered only when they involve intrusion into the solitude of individuals. The truly autonomous individual is assumed to exist, in a state of rationality or competence. The psychological nature of competence or the complexity associated with identifying the ends or purposes that competence instrumentally serves is frequently set aside. In fact, the empirical concreteness of the individual is nowhere to be found. Instead, the view becomes, as Thomas Nagel (1986) so aptly expressed it, the *view from nowhere*.

Finally, the emphasis on rights focuses attention on actions such as the delivery of goods and services that are either strictly forbidden or required. The domain of ethics is thus constricted; actions that are ethically permissible, including much of the domain of virtue, are viewed as having only peripheral relevance. Because they are not proscribed or required as a matter of right, such actions are of little interest. Yet if the central concern guiding long-term care involves caring for frail or dependent elders, it would seem that the focus should be on what is ethically optimal, not simply what is proscribed. Many things are ethically good that are not obligatory as a matter of someone's possession of a valid right. A child may not have a right to his parents' love, but only their care, yet the bestowal of love is surely ethically important nonetheless.

Limitations of rights

In Kantian terms, rights involve *perfect duties*, duties that are strict and determinate: perfect duties justify enforcement, that is, morally justify forcing others to honor the right possessed. This means that moral judgment, the concrete weighing of circumstances and considering the actual concrete existential situation, is hardly encouraged. Instead, morality is thought to consist in simply honoring valid rights claims no matter whether doing so conflicts with other moral goods or other values. Actions such as caring, compassion, or solicitude are relegated to a less significant or, indeed, a peripheral status. In general, what Kant termed *imperfect duties*, that is, duties that we all have as moral agents, such as the duty to be charitable or to be compassionate, are ignored. They are ignored precisely because they cannot be enforced as a matter of right. One cannot force someone to be compassionate. Instead, one must educate or develop the traits essential for the kind of caregiving that one wants to see in relationships such as parent–child or doctor–patient. Similarly, though charity is a general (imperfect) duty, it is indeterminate. Each of us is obliged to be charitable, but the obligation of charity does not carry with it any specification of the precise actions or circumstances that satisfy it. There is a range of discretion for judgment in the choice of actions and circumstances. To be sure, each of us reveals character traits and ideals in our choices and these are proper matters for ethical analysis and discussion, but our charitable actions are not corollaries of anyone's entitlement.

Rights language implicitly treats individuals in contractual (based on explicit agreement) or quasi-contractual (based on assumed or implicit agreement) terms and human relationships are generally defined in static and impersonal terms. Mary Ann Glendon (1993) has argued that even in the realm of the political, the dominance of rights language has led to an impoverishment of discourse, so it should not be surprising that rights language similarly impoverishes ethical discourse and discussion. As a result, a concept as complex and as rich as respect for persons is reduced to the formula of respecting the *rights* of individuals regarded abstractly. Persons are respected from an emotional and ethical distance. Real, actual individuals with life histories and personal experiences and stories are simply nowhere to be found! An implication of this view is that ethics comes down to ordering, weighing, or reconciling different values or interests. Hence, it should not surprise anyone to recognize that ethics has adopted available models for conducting such ordering and weighing from economics. The utilitarian calculus and contemporary applications of decision analysis have their roots in economic thinking. Indeed, the original sense of the term value and its cognate, worth, was monetary value. Only subsequently did the word take on the sense of the goodness of something. In the modern world, metaphors drawn from economics dominate our thinking about questions of value so much that we may have difficulty in appreciating the respects in which ethical value has formal properties that are different from monetary value (Whitbeck 1985: 184–5).

It is easy to recognize the implications of this association. Within the framework of the liberal concept of autonomy, values can be ordered, sometimes quantified, and maximized, and decision making is thought to be eminently a rational process. Choice consists in the weighing of values and preferences that individuals have. Asking whether the values and preferences that are morally worth having are independent of the quantitatively inspired sense of monetary value is an issue that makes little sense in this setting. Accordingly, ethics becomes involved with the task of discovering the rules that maximize the good or finding the fairest tradeoff among competing values. As a result, appeals to autonomy usually take two forms. First, those who are autonomous are allowed to make health care decisions for themselves free of undue influence or limitations, because their right to do so trumps all other considerations (Dworkin 1977). Second, those who do not possess the qualities of autonomy (such as those who are severely dependent, sick, or debilitated) are legitimately subject to decisions made on their behalf by surrogate decision makers.

It is interesting, and perhaps ironic, that surrogate decision making has assumed such importance in health care decisions (Buchanan and Brock 1989), but it is not surprising given the influence of legalistic thinking in medical ethics. On the liberal model of autonomy, individuals must possess minimal communication skills, minimal evidence of rationality, and minimum ability to comprehend the realities of their personal and social situation. Unfortunately, these requirements are infrequently met in medicine, particularly not in individuals requiring institutional long-term care. Since autonomy is the central and dominant concept that defines what medical ethics is, the alternatives are limited. A myth or fiction of decision making (hypothetically) by the patient is created to fill the void. Surrogate decision making thus carries the concept of autonomy as negative freedom to its logical conclusion: if individuals are, as autonomy seems to require, centers of impersonal, rational decision making, then such decision making can, indeed must, be exercised by others when the individuals cannot do so themselves. The only compelling question is really a procedural question, namely, who has the authority to exercise decision making for another? Because of our deep suspicion of physicians and other health care providers, the consensus response is anyone closely situated to the patient, so long as it is not the physician or health care provider. Some, rightly, have found the logic of surrogate decision making problematic (Buchanan 1983). At the very least, it is paradoxical and the paradox points to a systemic problem associated with the traditional view of autonomy as negative freedom, namely, that it assumes a rather abstract view of human persons. Before engaging that point, it will be useful to discuss a concern that is almost synonymous with the treatment of autonomy, that is, the problem of paternalism.

Paternalism and the development of persons

Although paternalism is a highly problematic term conveying extremely pejorative connotations, it has roots in a positive and essential feature of human development, namely, the parental nurturance of infants and children. Typical treatments of paternalism have not taken this connection seriously (exceptions include Douglas 1983; O'Neill 1984; Whitbeck 1985). In part, this is so because discussions of paternalism are so strikingly influenced by the liberal concept of autonomy. Another factor, however, complicates the discussion of paternalism in health care. Frequently, actions that are best described as beneficent, namely, actions undertaken without coercion to benefit a patient, are tarred with the brush of paternalism on the assumption that any action taken by a health care professional must in some objectionable way involve the imposition of professional power (Thomasma 1984: 911–12; Whitbeck 1985: 181). This is both understandable and lamentable.

So-called agency ethics or professional medical ethics defines the primary obligation of the physician to do everything possible to enhance the patient's welfare (American College of Physians 1984b: 266; Beauchamp and Childress 1983: 213; Daniels 1986: 1382; Fried 1978: 234; Judicial Council of the American Medical Association 1984: 3; Levinsky 1984: 1573; Pellegrino and Thomasma 1981: 275; Veatch 1981: 287). Indeed, some argue that concern for the patient's well-being or concern for justice is a more plausible foundation for medical ethics than autonomy (Childress 1990; Pellegrino and Thomasma 1988). Of course, it is not the only fundamental principle, as even defenders of professional medical ethics point out; the obligation to heal or benefit the patient acquires 'a normative force only when both physician and patients rank health and healing as primary' (Pellegrino and Thomasma 1981: 187). Nevertheless, the appeal to agency ethics and to the professional obligation of beneficence is frequently advanced in the service of political ends – for example debate over the introduction of procompetition and prospective payment into medicine. This line of argument misunderstands both the meaning and scope of a professional obligation of beneficence and the relationship between incentives and obligations (Agich 1986, 1987, 1990a, 1990b).

In light of these confusions and rhetorical ends to which appeal to the obligation of beneficence has been put, it is understandable that others have insisted that respect for persons and autonomy constitutes the only defensible secular and nonsectarian foundation for bioethics (Engelhardt 1986, 1991, 1997). The prominence given to the obligation of beneficence, of course, does not alone explain the counter-appeal of autonomy, but it is true that the most effective defense of patient autonomy and rights is firmly anchored in the analysis of power and authority. The fact that such debates continue clearly shows that the aim of subordinating autonomy to beneficence remains controversial.

Despite the overriding regard for self-determination promoted by the concept of autonomy just discussed, it has been recognized that there are possible moral justifications for departing from strict adherence to the rule of noninterference. As mentioned above, the inability of individuals to exhibit even minimal evidence of decision-making capacity makes the demand to respect autonomy – which means respecting an independent decision-making capacity – moot. In addition, the recognition of the basic facts of human development provides a ready, if only inadequately appreciated, basis for overriding autonomy. The fact is that human beings are not all-at-once persons, but develop historically as biopsychosocial entities under the care of human parents. This care, necessary for human growth and development, importantly includes interventions and actions that seem to constrain the infant's desires and actions, or otherwise interfere with self-determination. This fact is evident even to the staunchest individualist. Parental care is not only necessary for the development of human persons, but also provides a basis for morally justifying actions that limit or hinder the self-determination of another for that person's own good. Such acts are often labeled paternalistic.

Caroline Whitbeck (1985: 183) noted that most treatments of paternalism overlook this significant reference to human development and the dynamics of the relationship in which it occurs. In fact, most treatments are modeled on the role of the monarch in governing subjects, a role that is directed not toward making subjects into future monarchs but toward ensuring their survival and prosperity as subjects. She noted that this model can be traced at least to Aristotle and that it remarkably fails to include many of the central features of the parenting role. The focus instead is on the political relation of monarch to subject; no wonder, then, that the main concern is that of noninterference.

It is unfortunate that the sexist term paternalism has taken on such negative associations. Given the development of treatments of the parent–child relationship modeled on that of the monarch–subject from Aristotle onward, it is easy to see how public interactions shape the model that evolved. Unfortunately, the parent–child relationship is a relationship of intimacy in which paternal authority itself is a positive role that is certainly complemented by the nurturing, maternal role, but is in no way fundamentally opposed to it. If we have learned anything from empirical studies of childrearing practices, it is that these essential functions can be enacted in various ways. Some involve delineation along typical (for Western thought and experience) sex-determined parenting roles, but there is no logical requirement that such be the case. Recent experience of American families with two working parents has led to a variety of seemingly novel adaptations. It is common in professional couples, for instance, for the sex-delineated maternal and paternal roles to undergo dynamic adjustment as careers unfold and the child matures. Furthermore, common sense tells us that parents of either sex in the actual dynamic relations that constitute childrearing necessarily exercise parental authority and nurturance. Philosophers should be especially skeptical of stereotyped and static models. We must be careful not to speak of paternal authority and maternal nurturance as if they were sex-determined, mutually exclusive functions.

The concept of paternalism derives from the Latin *pater* because the fatherly role typically consists in protecting the children from harm and danger; the father does for the children what they cannot do for themselves, including interfering to restrict expressions of freedom that pose danger or risk of harm. The maternal role, on the other hand, is usually seen as nurturing. The mother nurtures the child from a state of total dependence to a state of increasing independence and responsibility. It is an active calling forth of the child, a positive role of facilitating development of the child's autonomy. The father figure is associated with authority, the mother with affection. The former is a restraining influence, the latter a liberating influence. Both, however, are essential components of parenting.

The question of the priority of the maternal or paternal role has surfaced in controversy over models of moral reasoning (Kittay and Meyers 1987). Lawrence Kohlberg (1971) proposed three levels of moral reasoning, each composed of two stages, moving from premoral to mature moral reasoning. Mature moral reasoning is illustrated by deontological reasoning, namely, the appeal to universal moral principles or roles that govern human action by respecting another person's rights. Carol Gilligan (1982, 1987), however, criticized Kohlberg's research because it is exclusively on the experience of males. Her research on female subjects yields a different model of responsibility or relationship that is not predicated on individual rights. Both models, however, seem prone to misuse. Kohlberg's categories, for example, were claimed to be applicable to all individuals (Rest et al. 1974) and Gilligan's work has been interpreted as arguing for the superiority of the female model (Saxton 1981), though there seems good reason to view each one as complementary to the other (Mahowald 1987: 24). Failure to appreciate complementary, yet dynamic, interrelationship between these models yields a remarkably one-sided view of ethics.

The term *parentalism* has been proposed as a nonsexist substitute for the term *paternalism* (Benjamin and Curtis 1981: 48–58). Others have objected that the substitution of the neutral term of parenting fails to overcome the sexist implications of paternal and maternal roles and ignores the real contributions of women that are irreplaceable by men. Mary B. Mahowald, however, argued that these concerns are valid only as a critique of a narrow notion of parenting and family relationships that prevail in today's society. The narrow notion views parenting as either maternally or paternally accomplished by individuals, as taking place merely during the period in which children are chronically young, and as occurring in a relationship that is biologically parental or legally adoptive (1987: 28–9). People who are not biological parents sometimes practice real parenting and biological parents sometimes miserably fail to fulfill the parental role. Parenting promotes autonomy of the other person even beyond the point where the nurturer's interventions are needed or desirable (Mahowald 1987: 29). Because parenting involves both life-begetting and life-sustaining functions, it involves an understanding of human life as an unfolding and developing process whose goal is the fulfillment of each individual's unique potential. Thus, parentalism is an apt term for a range of relationships that aim at enhancing the well-being of the lesser individual. The middle-aged woman who cares for her elderly senile father assumes the role of parent, by providing for his fundamental needs (the paternal role of protection) while encouraging as much autonomy as he is able to handle (the maternal role of nurturance).

When a balance exists between the roles of nurturance and protection, the ideal parenting is achieved. For this reason, the term *parentalism* can be used for a wide range of relationships that foster human development. Rather than making parentalism a nonsexist term for paternalism, parentalism should be used to express the complex positive meanings associated with the relationships that foster the development of persons. The pejorative term paternalism betrays a singular insensitivity to the positive significance of parenting in human development. As Thomas Halper observed:

'Paternalism' typically is greeted with all the enthusiasm reserved for a dead mouse in a dustpan. So powerful, in fact, are the word's pejorative connotations that in common speech it performs double duty: it describes a phenomenon and signals our distaste for it, both at the same time. However, this apparent economy is very costly, and the price is paid in terms of the vagueness, ambiguity, unexamined assumptions, and confusion. (1978: 331)

It seems evident to a degree that makes argument unnecessary that the life situation of most people is seldom one of total dependence or total independence. Many people are candidates for both protective and nurturing influences at various stages in their lives. People have needs that require attention and capabilities that need support. Moreover, the sequence of development is such that, even as adults, we may sometimes be more dependent than independent in our interdependence. As R.M. Hare (1972: 72–8) pointed out, the tension between protecting and nurturing is a false dichotomy or dilemma, because the dynamic relation between decisions and principles that are involved in actual moral life precludes any elevation of protection or nurturance above the other. Hare drew a rather interesting and important conclusion from this observation:

Many of the dark places of ethics become clear when we consider this dilemma in which parents are liable to find themselves. We have already noticed that, although principles have in the end to rest upon decisions of principle, decisions as such cannot be taught; only principles can be taught. It is the powerlessness of the parent to make for his son those many decisions of principle which the son during his future career will make, that gives moral language its characteristic shape. The only instrument which the parent possesses is moral education – the teaching of principles by example and precept, backed up by chastisement and other more up-to-date psychological methods. (1972: 75)

Hare also discussed the further dilemma that arises when moral education is primarily in terms of a fundamental choice between teaching principles or actual decision making. He argued that the dilemma posed by these two extreme alternatives is plainly false. Clearly, said Hare, you must provide children with a solid basis of principles at the same time that you afford ample opportunity for making decisions on which those principles are based and by which they are modified, improved, adapted to changed circumstances, or even abandoned if they are found to be unsuited to new situations (1972: 76). There is no dichotomy between principles and decisions. Rather, there is a dynamic relationship that is misunderstood if we exclusively concentrate on one or the other.

The parent–child situation nonetheless does seem to provide one significant model for justifying departures from the rule of noninterference; yet, as Whitbeck argued, the developmental context and the dynamic character of the relationship governing parent–child interactions were necessarily excluded from consideration of the assumptions underlying the liberal concept of autonomy (1985: 184). To rehabilitate the concept of autonomy as a guiding principle for long-term care thus requires an exploration of how persons actually develop and how ethical theory can accommodate actual autonomy.

From paternalism to parentalism

David Thomasma argued that acting in the best interests of another person means acting with respect for the other's personal independence and judgment (Thomasma 1984: 911). In so doing, autonomy is not waived. In health care contexts, illness and incapacity themselves impede freedom, so acting in another's best interests when they are ill need not be paternalistic. Some go so far as to assert that 'in theory the benefit principle assumes the waiving of autonomy' (Gadow 1980: 680), though no compelling argument has shown that this is the case. The tendency to shift from a consideration of beneficence (namely, acting to benefit the other or pursue the other's well-being) to a consideration of paternalism (namely, the imposition of a view of what constitutes the good for another against that other's own wishes) is a common enough mistake (Thomasma 1984: 911–12). In the case of dependent elders, Thomasma argued, illness and disability have already effaced the ability of the elder to choose independently; hence, the appropriate criterion is that 'the greater the dependence of the patient on others, the greater is the care that must be taken to act to enhance her well-being' (1984: 911).

An analogous point is captured in the distinction between direct and delegated autonomy (Collopy 1988). *Direct autonomy* involves explicit decision making and action by an individual, independent agent; *delegated autonomy* involves the acceptance or authorization of actions and decisions by others for oneself. In some contexts, delegated autonomy can surely be seen as a loss of autonomy, but for frail elders delegated autonomy can actually extend autonomy and independence. To argue that delegation is wrong means that one should be willing to impose on a frail elder the full weight of her unsupported independence. The concept of delegated autonomy directs attention to the unique ethical character of long-term care and suggests the need for an independent assessment of its reality where there is a dynamic interplay between competence and incompetence, control and freedom (Collopy 1988: 12; May 1982).

This response is often characterized as paternalism, but it might better be described as *parentalism*, that is, the situation in which an affectively concerned caregiver strives to enhance the well-being, including the autonomy, of another dependent individual. In effect, parentalism would be the better term for what has been called *autonomy-respecting paternalism* (VanDeVeer 1986). Parentalism assumes that the caregiver does not cause the dependence and that the caregiver, through any form of coercion, does not sustain it. It also assumes that the caregiver's view of the dependent individual's well-being is not imposed over the free and competent choice of the dependent other.

Parentalism has its roots in a phenomenon essential to being a human person, namely, that a human person does not spring into being fully formed as an independent agent but develops through psychosocial relations with human parents. Parentalism signals the essential interconnectedness of all human persons and is rooted in the basic response to the needy other that such relationships engender. Parentalism also points to the fact that adult human beings are necessarily interdependent and, despite their maturity, require nurturance. They exist as persons through action in the common and shared world of everyday life. The problem of autonomy is wrongly characterized if it is simply juxtaposed to paternalism. Mill's important reflections in *On Liberty* (1978) occur under the simplifying assumption that the agent is in the full maturity of her faculties. That assumption is unquestioned in liberal thought, but it is equally unsupportable in long-term care. For that reason, a full account of what it means to be a human person is required to adequately understand what autonomy means in long-term care. We are concerned, after all, with autonomy not theoretically, but with the reality of the conditions of loss and dependence that bring individuals into long-term care.

One might certainly object that parentalism is nothing more than a semantic sleight of hand, because the position is the same as weak paternalism, namely, that it justifies actions undertaken against unreasonable or incompetent decision making. True enough, but weak paternalism typically focuses on the cognitive and volitional capacities that comprise human autonomy, leaving aside the affective, conative, and communicative aspects that parentalism is better able to accommodate.

These points, of course, do not resolve the issue of paternalism. Paternalism is not likely to be so easily dismissed. It remains a lively issue, because two questionable assumptions that are central to liberal theory permeate its construction: first, that individuals are by definition (and so in reality) fully capable of rational, free choice, and second, that paternalism is as much a compelling practical concern in everyday life as it is in theory. The first assumption is questionable insofar as it rests on an abstract and somewhat naive view of the phenomenon of autonomy. The second assumption is questionable insofar as it rests on thin assessment of actual phenomena of autonomous action and choice. In many standard discussions of paternalism, autonomy is treated entirely in formal or abstract terms due to the general tendency of contemporary ethics to consider only contrived cases or examples.

To rectify this situation, it will be necessary to engage in what Clifford Geertz (1973, 1984) called *thick description*, a description that is attentive to the fullest concrete circumstances that comprise the subject under discussion. Such an approach is facilitated by methodologically setting aside our theoretical prejudices about autonomy. Under these circumstances, ethics might prove to be relevant to those nettlesome complexities of everyday life that are otherwise overlooked (Kane and Caplan 1990). Consequently, ethical reflection will have to become more empirical and phenomenological on the one hand and far more practical and pragmatic on the other. An engagement with involvement in the everyday world of long-term care is unfortunately lacking in the so-called applied field of bioethics. The issue of paternalism represents a formidable obstacle to an ethics of long-term care, because it resides at a level at least once removed from the mundane experience of care. Once autonomy and long-term care are seen in their ordinary and everyday settings, we will more readily appreciate why parentalism is a more apt characterization of the phenomena. The traditional problem of paternalism as a counterpoint to liberty is thus not solved by our approach, so much as it is transformed from a theoretical quandary into a practical dialectic animated by what Ronald Dworkin (1977: 272–3) calls concern and respect.

Summary

Liberalism and the liberal view of autonomy are defensible when confined to the political/legal order. Within that realm, autonomy is an indisputably important value, though it may not be the primary value even there. The political/legal realm, however, is not coextensive with human life and certainly does not exhaust the realm of ethics. The political/legal concept of autonomy primarily concerns the relationship of individuals and the state and, by extension, the public interactions in our complex multifaceted society. It only partly defines other aspects of social existence, such as the interactions between intimates of various sorts. Hence, the liberal theory of autonomy and the view of persons that it entails are not an adequate account of autonomy. Autonomy is a far more complex phenomenon than is routinely appreciated in the standard accounts inspired by liberal theory. Even though worries over paternalism naturally flow from a view of autonomy in which independence and noninterference are primary values, in health care failures of communication on the part of the health professional are more prominent than paternalistic behaviors. As Whitbeck observed, physicians seldom display truly paternalistic behavior toward patients; they act beneficently (Whitbeck 1985: 181). Behavior can properly be described as paternalistic only if it results from a decision to override the autonomous choice of patients, but physicians and other health care workers seldom make such judgments. They often simply fail to communicate effectively with patients on matters that are troubling to them, especially involving matters of dying or uncertainty. Thus, the problem of paternalism should not distract us any further from attending to the actual complexities associated with manifestations of autonomy in long-term care. Human beings develop and express their autonomy in a social world that is complex. In fact, human beings attain autonomy only through human relationships and the exercise of autonomy requires supportive relationships throughout one's life. Hence, we need to consider more fully the reality of human development and relationships within which autonomy actually operates.

3

Long-term care: myth and reality

Discussion of autonomy in long-term care is complicated because assumptions about the nature of caregiving relationships provide inaccurate, inadequate, and misleading models for long-term care. Long-term care is often assumed to be institutional care in which elders live without familial or other social supports. The ethical problem is seen in this institutional context as involving conflicts over basic rights as the long-term care *total institution* (Goffman 1960, 1961) strips elders of self-control and self-respect. The empirical evidence, however, presents a more complicated picture that seems to belie the values of independence and the right of noninterference that are at the core of the bioethical response.

Survey data demonstrate that over 70 percent of home care is delivered by family and friends, not paid providers (Rabin and Stockton 1987: 151), a percentage that parallels the 67 percent of older noninstitutionalized persons who lived in a family setting in 1998 (Administration on Aging 2000). Families contributed financially to the institutional care of older relatives and 13 percent of older persons (7 percent of men and 17 percent of women) were living with children, siblings, or relatives other than a spouse (Administration on Aging 2000). Instead of the picture of isolated, vulnerable old people needing the protection from an impersonal institution, a picture emerges in which the majority of dependent old people maintain various kinds of integrated lives, often in proximity to family and friends. The received view is that long-term care is predominantly impersonal, institutional, and medical, whereas it involves a spectrum of caregiving from family to professional in a variety of settings. This chapter, however, is focused less on data about actual long-term care than on the mythology associated with being old and frail that shapes our thinking about the meaning of autonomy in long-term care. Cultural prejudices about being old are reinforced by the dominant model of care in our society based on acute care. To speak of mythology is not to speak of false beliefs, since myths are not contrary to reality or truth; instead, myths are deep-seated, tacit beliefs that reflect the basic frames of meaning and interpretation in any society.

Myths of old age

Simone de Beauvoir noted that the old are invisible because we see death with a clearer eye than old age itself (1972: 4). She means that because the aged are close to death, we look beyond them at the fearful prospect of our own demise, thereby marginalizing their existence. The way that younger and healthier people perceive elders affects the way that they behave toward elders. Empirical evidence suggests that these modes of perception are socially influenced, if not socially determined, so it is not surprising that social ideas about autonomy are expressed here. Becoming aware of the mythology and metaphors associated with being old can help us understand the ways that our own interactions with – or avoidances of – elders reflect latent prejudices that need to be exposed if their ethical status is to be assessed.

Old age is typically regarded as a life-stage predominantly characterized by loss of capacity. The effacement of the autonomy of elders takes many forms, but the process of devaluation clearly does not occur only in the individual; it is a product of assumptions about being old in our society. Uncovering these assumptions is exceedingly difficult. It is sometimes thought that the loss of autonomy is related to the institutionalization that inevitably segregates elders from society, but perhaps a truer interpretation is that the phenomenon of nursing home care in America itself reflects diffuse social attitudes and values about being old, though nursing homes undoubtedly contribute to these attitudes in a kind of unrelenting chain reaction. We can identify the main elements of this stereotype by selectively reviewing the literature on the meaning and cultural significance of old age.

A good place to begin is the concept expressed by Rosalie Rosenfelt under the title 'The elderly mystique' (1965). Core to the concept of the elderly mystique is the sense that the old person herself explicitly expects derogation. The elderly mystique simply holds that the potential for continuing engagement, development, and growth virtually disappears in elders, especially when disabled. A consequence of this mystique is that both professional and family caregivers focus on maintaining activities of daily living and keeping the elderly person out of a nursing home, which encourages her to perceive herself as having little or no choice and she experiences a diminished sense of her own autonomy (Cohen 1988: 24). The elderly mystique seems to be an outgrowth of the phenomenon originally termed ageism by Butler (1975).

Ageism is a process involving the systematic stereotyping of and discrimination against people just because they are old, as racism and sexism do with skin color and gender. Old people are categorized as senile, rigid in thought and manner, and old-fashioned in morality and skills. Ageism allows younger generations to see older people as fundamentally different from themselves, so they subtly cease to identify with their elders as human beings (Butler 1975). Ageism originally described the pejorative cultural attitudes and beliefs about elders that seemed to become a dominant social theme after World War II, though now it appears to focus less on elders than on elders with disabilities (Cohen 1988: 25). Elders themselves seem to share the view that when a disability arrives, hope about growth, self-realization, or participation with family and society must be abandoned so that all personal energy can be directed toward avoiding 'the ultimate defeat, which is not death but institutionalization which is regarded as a living death' (Cohen 1988: 25).

Charles Taylor (1979) suggested that there is a new ageism that is particularly prominent in advocates for elders who stereotypically view all elders in terms of a kind of least common denominator, namely, in terms of those who are least capable, least healthy, and least alert, so that elders as a class are seen as helpless and dependent individuals who require a variety of specialized support services. The development of these services is encouraged with unbridled enthusiasm and without much concern regarding how these services might reduce the freedom of elders to make decisions about their own lives. This enthusiasm may be guided by beneficent motives, but its underlying premise is surely suspect, since the definition of needs and the determination of the kinds of services that adequately meet these needs are usually made by professionals, not the elders themselves. These paternalistic attitudes pose a clear threat to autonomy, especially for disabled and frail elders who are the most likely recipients of these beneficent intentions and the least capable of resisting the proffered help.

The negative attitudes toward old age, especially toward disabled elders, is a corollary of the stress on individualism in the literature on aging, a stress that seems, in part, to be a projection of the standards of middle-aged behavior onto old people, in which activity and independence function as tacit norms. There appears a latent assumption that successful aging consists in being as much like a middle-aged person as possible. This means that feeling useful is especially important, even though feeling useful has been left undefined. Apparently because the values of middle age are so tacit, this literature does not make it clear why old people should be expected to feel that way (Havighurst 1956: 54–5). If one cannot satisfy these norms, then that deviance must be explained. A good example of this kind of explanation is the disengagement theory of aging:

Starting from the common-sense observation that the old person is less involved in the life around him than he was when he was younger, we can describe the process by which he becomes so, and we can do this without assumptions about its desirability. In our theory, aging is an inevitable mutual withdrawal or disengagement, resulting in decreased interaction between the aging person and others in the social systems he belongs to. His withdrawal may be accompanied at the outset by an increased preoccupation with himself; certain institutions in society may make this withdrawal easy for him. When the aging process is complete, the equilibrium which existed in middle life between the individual and his society has given way to a new equilibrium characterized by a greater distance and an altered type of relationship. (Cumming and Henry 1961: 14–15)

Thomas Cole (1985) pointed out that in our society a significant gulf separates age and youth, a gulf that is manifest in the bureaucratized social life course, the psychological life of individuals, and in the collective imagination of popular culture. When age and youth are fractured into polarities, a self-destructive cycle evolves. Pointing to progress in the material and physical conditions of life for elders in the late twentieth century does not erase the great spiritual and ethical price that has been paid. A society that values productivity and material wealth above other values is understandably youth oriented; a natural consequence is that the old come to be seen, and to see themselves, as obsolete and redundant. The polarization of youth and old age is significant despite advances in the material welfare of elders. One cannot conclude that a personally meaningful sense of security or dignity in old age is attained just because Social Security and other social programs for the old are in place (Christiansen 1978). In fact, elders continue to occupy a marginal status in society despite their improved economic status for the simple reason that the fundamental social values are wrapped up in a commitment to grow without limit (Cole 1985: 51). As a result, elders are estranged from the main cultural and social forces; they are marginalized not only by the actions of others, actions that might as particular behaviors be quite caring and understanding, but also by the value system that makes up our social fabric.

To take elders seriously as full autonomous moral agents, then, must involve, more than acknowledging or advocating for their independence or entitlement to social services. It means according them full status in everyday social life. Beyond invoking the principle of autonomy against the paternalism of health professionals or establishing a list of elder rights, understanding the responsibilities or obligations of elders as well as the virtues that age calls for is needed (Jameton 1988; May 1986). Such considerations, however, are seldom prominent concerns. In a sense this is understandable, since the aging industry, including the academic and professional gerontological component, is itself a cultural response to the problem of being old in a society that prizes youth and productivity. Interpreting the ethical problems associated with long-term care in terms of the culturally prominent ideal of independence reflects taken-for-granted beliefs that mirror the public policy response to old age in terms of economic, health care, housing, or social services. Nevertheless, the fact remains that the underlying paradox or tension associated with autonomy and long-term care is hardly relieved by such a strategy. For example, the problem of providing adequate health care for our entire population has come up against the social commitments to the aged as a class needing special attention. The resulting problems of setting limits (Callahan 1987) and the resulting issues of intergenerational justice (Daniels 1988) reflect not only cultural confusion about the meaning of old age, but also life-span development (Agich 2001).

Both negative stereotypes of elders as dependent individuals who need costly and specialized services and who are incapable of leading real lives and are simply an economic drain on society, as well as positive images of elders who are active, healthy, and engaged in their special retirement lifestyles reflect a cultural pattern in which elders are generally regarded as outside the social mainstream or are otherwise culturally isolated (Francher 1969). Some authors suggest that this cultural pattern has been reinforced by the growth of segregated institutions for the aged (Dowd 1985; Gruman 1978), but the deeper question is the symbolic meaning and cultural values that are latent in the isolated status that is created for elders. Importantly, the old represent not only obsolescence or a devalued past, but also a future that no one wants, a future that can be repressed only if the elder is effectively alienated from the vision of one's own future self (Cole 1985). The image of the elder as other or stranger is an important cultural development that parallels cultural attitudes about deviants of all sorts who symbolically threaten fundamental beliefs and values central to the dominant sense of self (Gilman 1988). The earliest visions of the elder as a stranger in the modern period can be found in late eighteenth-century Romantic literature, but apparently did not become widespread until the growth of retirement (Graebner 1980) and the rise of an industry devoted to aging (Estes 1979). In a sense, efforts to endow elders with a significant social status that they can longer enjoy in a production-oriented and work-oriented society seem to have contributed to their isolation and have fostered the meaninglessness and despair that are commonly observed characteristics of old age.

Negative images of old age in the Western world are sometimes contrasted with other societies. Studies have shown that elders in other societies enjoy considerable respect and occupy important advisory and spiritual roles in family and community, for example among the Samoans (Holmes and Rhoads 1983), the Druze of Lebanon (Guttman 1976), the Japanese (Plath 1983), the Chinese (Harrell 1979), and many Native American tribes (Schweitzer 1983). The anthropological evidence, however, is not one sided. Other societies, such as the Shiriono of Bolivia (Holmberg 1969), the Tasmanians of the South Pacific (Roth 1890), and the Xosa of South Africa (Kidd 1904), are reported to abuse, neglect, or disparage the few old people living in their societies. It would thus be a mistake to conclude that cultures with more positive attitudes toward elders are the norm and that our Western society is deviant. The existence of societies that do exhibit positive attitudes and provide positive social roles for their elders supplies us with a set of ideals and shows us what is humanly possible; in doing so, these societies provide a lens that helps us see what is characteristic of our own society and historical period. As Savishinsky observed: 'The modern marginality of the old is a hallmark of the very first century to see the elderly become a sizable, problematic portion of the population, with ill-defined roles and responsibilities' (1991: 2).

The picture of old age is thus exceedingly complex, because there does not seem to be a single social response to old age and because the meaning of being old is surrounded by cultural beliefs and values that are central to our contemporary social life. Generally, evidence suggests that elders are doing well in retirement, despite beliefs held by the medical community and lay people that retirement has an adverse impact on health status (Portnoi 1981). Attitudes among elders toward old age and retirement, such as the images of robustly active retirees normatively projected by groups like the American Association of Retired Persons (AARP), strongly shade the picture. Elders do live in their own homes or apartments, retirement communities, senior citizens' housing complexes, as well as nursing homes. Some are steeped in an ethnic identity and others are devoid of such a heritage. The class of *the elderly* includes both the rich and poor, sick and well, sane and insane; it also embraces the relatively healthy so-called *young old* between 60 and 75 and the more vulnerable *old old* who are living beyond their eighth decade. Some are intimately connected with family and community, whereas others are cut off from their kin. Some are active and ardent; others are disengaged and hopeless (Savishinsky 1991: 2). The picture is probably best described as a collage composed of both complementary and dissonant images. The surest thing to say about old age in the Western world is that it defies easy generalization. Why that is the case is certainly complex, but is rooted in cultural meanings that test and taunt the dominant vision of the person as an independent, active, and productive individual competently negotiating the everyday world.

Nursing homes

The mythology of old age is important because it shapes the Western understanding of autonomy and provides a backdrop for any treatment of long-term care. While the causal relations between long-term care and attitudes toward old age are speculative at best, there are parallels between the two that help us understand why autonomy is a uniquely relevant problem. As discussed in Chapter 1, long-term care is frequently represented in various icons of nursing home life. These icons of nursing home existence express basic anxiety about long-term care that bears directly on the meaning of autonomy itself.

Researchers have identified clear ambiguities and strains in institutional care: for example, some staff think of the institution as a home whereas others see it as a hospital (Shield 1988); some staff members emphasize humanitarian ideals of care while their colleagues stress cure (Vesperi 1983); and there are pronounced tensions between those who follow a social as opposed to a medical model of treatment (Kane and Kane 1978). One point, however, is clear, namely, that many individuals view old age as joyless and terrible and feel that nursing homes only make matters worse.

Such institutions are seen as the last resort of those who can no longer help themselves. In the apparent uselessness of one's later years, they symbolize rejection, and they sometimes rub the salt of neglect into the moral wounds of marginality. This sad, spoiled image of late life contrasts with the equally extreme myth of the golden age of old age, a once hallowed but now suspect truth that people no longer believe in. The imagination of our culture has transformed the old dream into a new nightmare. (Savishinsky 1991: 1)

The overriding theme of the literature on the nursing home experience is one of rejection and loss. In light of this vision of long-term care, one might say of our society what William Butler Yeats said of Byzantium: 'That is no country for old men' (1959: 191). The message of much of the literature is that elders, too, find the world of the nursing home to be foreign and forbidding. Unable to manage in the outside world that is inhospitable and unsupportive of their unique needs, they experience the nursing home as a kind of purgatory or limbo, a fate almost worse than death. The titles of some of this literature are remarkably revealing: *A Home is Not a Home* (Tulloch 1975), *Tender Loving Greed* (Mendelson 1975), *Why Survive?* (Butler 1975), *Unloving Care* (Vladeck 1980), *Nobody Ever Died of Old Age* (Curtin 1972), *Old Age: The Last Segregation* (Townsend 1971), *Sans Everything* (Robb 1968), *Uneasy Endings* (Shield 1988), *The Ends of Time* (Savishinsky 1991) and *the Erosion of Autonomy in Long-Term Care* (Lidz, Fisher, and Arnold 1992).

One of the more personal reports of nursing home life was provided by Carobeth Laird, an anthropologist who at the age of 79 was placed in an Arizona geriatric facility. After her discharge several months later when friends learned of her plight and offered a place to live, she wrote a book entitled *Limbo: A Memoir of Life in a Nursing Home by a Survivor* (1979). She described a number of experiences that are commonly reported for institutionalized elders: a profound loss of control over daily life, an overwhelming sense of isolation, a preoccupation with bodily functions such as eating and excretion, a sense of financial insecurity, a distortion of her own perception of reality and sense of time, and a loss of her sense of self-identity. These are recurrent observations in the nursing home literature that any account of autonomy and the nursing home experience needs to integrate. Although choice was evidently restricted for Laird, loss of choice as such was not the central concern. Other kinds of experience seem to be crucially significant for elders in nursing homes.

Maria Vesperi (1983) and Timothy Diamond (1986), who worked as aides in nursing homes, published intriguing ethnographic studies of everyday life in them. Their work provides a unique insight into everyday life in nursing homes from the primary caregiver perspective. Nursing assistants constitute one of the largest and fastest growing occupational groups in the United States. Although some men do the work, most nursing assistants are women. As Diamond reported, one of the most important things taught in the training course was not to ask questions or show initiative, but to do as one was told.

One of the students, a black woman from Jamaica, was reported to joke: 'I can't figure out whether they're trying to teach us to be nurses' aides or black women' (1986: 1287). Their daily work is defined mainly in terms of helping elders with sensory and cognitive impairment to complete activities of daily living (ADLs).

Like the majority of elders in nursing homes, nurses' aides are usually female and often poor (Diamond 1986). They are predominantly nonwhite women, even though most owners and directors of nursing homes are white men. Their jobs are hard. Nursing assistants are overwhelmingly paid rates that are scandalously low; hence, the primary providers of care for institutionalized elders are, by any measure, an exploited population. Most nursing assistants are paid at a rate that creates poverty. Even working full-time, they earn less than family subsistence and many assistants are reported to work more than one job if they can or to live in hope of overtime (Diamond 1986: 1288). A society that measures worth and importance largely in monetary terms provides a harsh judgment about the esteem associated with this type of caregiving. Undoubtedly, this message reverberates in the day-to-day life of the nursing home. For example, frequent turnover of staff subjects elders to repeated adaptation that introduces a constant source of stress and anxiety into the daily lives of individuals whose coping abilities are compromised by cognitive or physical impairments.

Diamond reported that he brought a number of preconceptions about elders in long-term care to his work. For example, he thought of them as passive recipients of someone else's acts, as acted on rather than acting (1986: 1289). Admittedly, the nursing home residents are defined by the social structure and organization of nursing homes in a passive way; they are literally patients and not agents. They are named in terms of their diseases and their basic record of care, the chart, is about what is to be done to them, such as feeding, bathing, or toileting, not in terms of what they do. To outside observers, their existence appears remarkably passive; infrequent short visits provide snapshot images of people just sitting (Diamond 1986: 1289). Day rooms filled with a score of elders are typically bereft of conversation or other meaningful interactions. However, there is another side to the everyday reality of life in a nursing home that evades most casual observers, a reality that extends beyond these static pictures. Once one gets to know elders as individuals, it becomes clear that almost all are thinking and conscious people, though their consciousness might be fragile and intermittent and their concerns different from our own.

Diamond reports that elders actively participate in various nursing home activities. They are not simply acted upon, but struggle to maintain their own consciousness and identity, even if appearances belie this effort (Diamond 1986: 1290). If appearances do belie this effort, it is because we assume that real work is objectified in the world as a work, a product, or a material object produced by one's efforts. The concept of work is closely related to the

phenomena of pain and imagination; like them, it presses toward objectification, though the objectification is not always so evidently a physical thing in
the world (Scarry 1985). Rather, the primary work activities in which many
(particularly institutionalized) elders engage involves remaking the world for
experience, reconstituting the meaning structures for their lives, not simply
forming objects within the ambient world. Too often, the kind of effort required
for such world-making is overlooked, because standard accounts of autonomy
seldom adequately address the need for individuals to actively define or make
a world. Instead, standard accounts of autonomy focus instead on discrete
choices or decisions within a pre-given frame of reality or reference. One implication of these points is that any adequate account of autonomy in long-term
care needs to understand and make sense of the activity of world-making in
which even seemingly passive or confused elders unavoidably engage.

Although nursing home residents are not by definition passive, they are
remarkably dependent. The ability to perform ADLs such as dressing, grooming, bathing, or eating cannot safely be assumed for these individuals. In fact,
the job description of nurses' aides mainly involves assistance with the basic
functions of daily living such as helping individuals get in and out of bed,
giving baths, assisting elders in the toilet or in feeding. The 1985 National
Nursing Home Survey reported that 91 percent of residents needed help with
bathing, 75 percent with dressing, 63 percent with getting in and out of bed
or a chair, 40 percent with eating, and 50 percent experienced some bladder
or bowel incontinence (Hing 1987).

Coupled with the need for assistance in routine ADLs, most elders in nursing homes suffer from a variety of sensory and cognitive deficits: for example,
63 percent of all nursing home residents are demented or have serious memory impairments (Hing 1987). Although some caution should be exercised
in interpreting these data, since the diagnostic data are drawn from notation
in the residents' charts that often reflects assumptions rather than a serious
work-up (Kane 1990: 9), considerable cognitive impairment undoubtedly
exists in elders living in nursing homes. Some studies indicate that as many as
75 percent of nursing home residents have some degree of mental impairment
(Larsen, Lo, and Williams 1986). These data, however, do not necessarily mean
that autonomy is absent, though prejudices associated with mental illness or
deficits commonly involve the assumption that anyone who is mentally ill or
impaired is by definition incompetent. These facts cannot be overlooked in
conceptualizing autonomy in long-term care. Other findings, too, are relevant.
For example, after surveying 111 programs in a three-state area, Hegeman and
Tobin (1988) reported that the functioning of mentally impaired elders can be
improved through a wide range of interventions including special program-
ming like small group activities involving reminiscence, validation therapy,
discussion, and sensory stimulation; structural and environmental adaptations; and staff training and deployment. Even some of the most confused

residents can be helped to preserve their remaining identity and disoriented elders can be helped to be more oriented to time and place, thus providing them with some of the prerequisites for self-determination.

Studies of nursing homes, however, are rife with evidence that various common practices infantilize and depersonalize elders. These practices include not respecting the elder's privacy, restricting personal possessions or visitation, and not assuring reliable transportation or in-house services. Coupled with the need to adapt to the total environment of a nursing home that isolates, controls, and reconstitutes the daily lives of elders who live in them, these standard nursing home practices constitute impressive assaults on autonomy. Since staff are primarily oriented toward pursuing medically related activities – the dominant mode of discourse, the schedule, and evaluations are based on the performance of such specific tasks as bathing, feeding, or toilet assistance – the full effect of these practices on the autonomy of residents often goes unnoticed. The medically defined objectives rarely take into account that the elder is an experiencing subject and person. Instead, the elder is made the object of a style of care that functionally compromises the conditions needed to sustain autonomy.

Vesperi (1983) noted a fundamental contradiction between patient expectations and staff goals. The predominant training model for nurses' aides is a medical model. The education of nurses' aides and their daily work are defined in a task-centered, physical way (Diamond 1986: 1290). The day starts with staff members having to rouse patients, who invariably grumble at the early awakening times. Elders must be awakened, dressed, and prepared for breakfast and medications. They are then transported, if they are not bedfast, to the day room for breakfast. If the nurses' aide is stuck with too many *feeders*, namely, patients who need help eating, it proves impossible to finish breakfast at the appointed time. Coupled with the slow pace of many elders in eating, particularly those who dislike the food or are still not yet fully awake, the relentless rush of the scheduled close of breakfast creates anxiety for staff who are understandably disinclined to engage in any kind of meaningful interaction with their charges. Activities after breakfast, such as helping elders with showers or bed baths, toileting or bed pans, changing beds, taking vital signs, dealing with constant individual requests, and recording it all in the chart, keep the staff extremely busy until lunch, when the ordeal of the meal resumes.

Much of this activity is important and essential in the care of institutionalized elders, though it is often infused with meanings that are bizarre at best. Despite all the attention to physical well-being and the maintenance of the trappings of the hospital, such as uniforms, charts, and the recording of vital signs, there is little real therapeutic intent. The treatment simply does not aim toward any therapeutic objective, but is carried out at the level of custodial care. As Savishinsky reported, 'this lack of emphasis on restoring people's health defeated the best hopes of residents and intensified their tendency to decline' (1991: 6). The underlying problem is not only the way that restoring health or maintaining well-being is not pursued, but that there is significant confusion about the basic meaning of health or well-being for an institutionalized frail elder.

Even though nursing homes are not hospitals, they are medical environments. The trappings of the hospital are in evidence everywhere, from the chart, regular recording of the units of health care delivered, and the diagnosis or dominance of disease language in description of residents, to sanitized environment and the officiously busy and uniformed staff. Daily work is defined in a task-centered fashion focused on the provision of services associated with ADLs. Task responsibility is oriented toward the objective action to be performed rather than the recipient of the action (Agich 1982: 66). Such an orientation to responsibility in one's work thrives in a bureaucratic organization in which a hierarchical structure of authority promotes an external accountability for the caregiver's behavior rather than a subjective or internal accountability in terms of the caregiver's own judgment. This understanding of the basic responsibility of caregivers contributes to the feeling of estrangement and frustration that nurses' aides are reported to exhibit. The bureaucratic structure of the typical nursing home assures that supervisory staff, who are usually found to be well-removed from the actual caregiving, keeping records in offices or nursing stations, have little actual appreciation of what it takes for nurses' aides to accomplish daily work routines. They do not understand that the structure of daily work effectively thwarts any vestiges of autonomy in elders. Coupled with the low levels of pay and education, and the undeniable stress of work, direct-care staff members understandably display negative work attitudes, as evidenced by the high rate at which they resign (Diamond 1986: 1287–8; Savishinsky 1991: 5).

Although the nursing home is commonly viewed as a way station on the road to death, national data suggest a more complicated picture. There is good reason to assume that there are two separate streams of patients passing through nursing homes: a short-stay group whose average length of stay is approximately 1.9 months and a long-stay group who stay about 2.5 years. Although the latter group accounts for only 39 percent of discharges, they comprise 91 percent of the residents at any one time (Keeler, Kane, and Solomon 1981). Although nursing homes are prominent sites of long-term care for many elders, they are remarkably transient institutions. There is considerable coming and going as patients are discharged, reassigned to different units based on staff judgments about (among other things) the level and kind of care needed and new admissions. Coupled with staff turnover, an air of change, unreality, and rootlessness naturally emerges that undoubtedly creates stress and confusion for the residents. Despite the significance of these changes, residents typically have little or no say about the environment of change.

The make-up of nursing homes inevitably includes individuals with diverse educational, ethnic, occupational, religious, and social backgrounds as well as levels of income (Macklin 1990). They are anything but communities or homes. The lack of a sense of community is addressed in some institutions by the adopting of explicit rituals or practices intended to construct a sense of community, but often little or nothing is done to foster, or even to permit, meaningful relationships or associations to develop among the residents themselves. Indeed, assignment of roommates or rooms by staff, a commonplace occurrence in nursing homes, significantly limits resident autonomy (Miles and Sachs 1990).

Institutions that are church-run or that have a distinct ethnic or religious make-up surprisingly show the same anomie and meaningless characteristic of secular institutions. Jaber Gubrium (1975) observed that day-to-day routines centered on the cognitive organization of life and labor in a church-run institution he called Murray Manor. He described various structural divisions between top staff and floor staff, the dominant attention to bed and body work by floor staff, the ritual outings of residents, and the unique status enjoyed by those who received visitors, as well as the implicit and explicit ways that elders staked out personal space by claiming chairs or lounge areas. Gubrium also reported that administrators propounded an ethic of sensitive individualized care, but they stayed comfortably away from the everyday work world of floor staff so that they infrequently saw how patients were actually treated.

Mary O'Brien (1989) described Bethany Manor, a 230-bed east coast nursing home whose funding, supervisory staff, and elders were primarily drawn from the Catholic community. The facility's religious atmosphere and services seemed to help many residents develop and sustain an accepting attitude toward death, but other anxieties and fears associated with being old and frail were present nonetheless. There was, for instance, a significant fear of surviving with a lingering cognitive deficit (O'Brien 1989: 96) or being transferred to the skilled nursing floor, a fate that was viewed as worse than death (O'Brien 1989: 32).

Reneé Rose Shield (1988) similarly described a nonprofit Jewish facility located in a northeastern city. While residents shared a common religious background, the facility was not able to provide them with a sense of community or any effectively meaningful way to ease their transition to old age and impairment. Shield attributed these failures to several factors, including the controlling nature of institutional regulations, the inability of elders to reciprocate what others gave them, the tendency of elders to preserve their autonomy by remaining aloof from one another, and a lack of staff consensus regarding whether the facility was a home or a hospital. As a result, a variety of inequities and contradictions were expressed in institutional rules that tended to place residents and staff in adversarial relationships (Shield 1988: 22).

The picture of long-term care presented in the nursing home literature is clearly bleak. In the United States, this situation is in part attributable to the way that long-term care is funded as a health-related welfare benefit for the poor rather than a health benefit or social service for all. It is a matter of public policy that long-term care benefits depend on medical definitions of the need for care (Kane and Kane 1990: 86). Ironically, the more dependent people are, the more eligible they are for care based on their inability to perform specific basic activities such as ADLs and IADLs (instrumental activities of daily living). The result is a payment system that rewards dependency by creating disincentives to caregivers to help clients to recover or improve functioning. This payment system impedes or thwarts autonomy (Kane and Kane 1990: 86).

Part of the difficulty is the emphasis given to formal rehabilitation services that have as their goal maximizing the functional abilities of disabled and impaired elders over other care that is viewed as merely custodial. Since recovery of function is tied to reversible medical problems, other functional disabilities tend to be accepted as irremediable. Unless elders are formally eligible for a reimbursable rehabilitation program, they are not usually helped to improve their functioning. As a result, payment mechanisms actually limit the elders' choice about the place and type of care as well as constrain many daily choices that elders make. Ironically, elders with functional impairments sometimes only require the help of others to carry out their choices, so that autonomy may actually be restricted precisely when an elder's independence is respected. When elders require help to do things on their own, but that help is not available for reimbursement or bureaucratic reasons, positive autonomy is existentially compromised.

This point involves the distinction between decisional and executional autonomy (Collopy 1988). Decisional autonomy is the ability to make decisions without external restraint or coercion. Executional autonomy is the ability and freedom to act on decisional autonomy. For most individuals, autonomy is at once decisional and executional, but it need not always be so and individuals can be able to decide while lacking the ability or freedom to execute decisions. An implication of this distinction is that if autonomy is defined primarily by execution, then frail or confused elders will be, by definition, nonautonomous. However, because decisional autonomy can remain intact when executional autonomy wanes, failure to provide adequate help to an incapacitated elder can seriously efface autonomous choice. As Collopy noted, 'as the outward reach of autonomy shrinks, its inner decisional core becomes a last and therefore most crucial preserve of self-determination' (1988: 12). Supporting executional autonomy, then, is an important way to respect an elder's autonomy. Doing so, however, entails more than simply forbearance, because specific support needs to be positively provided.

Present nursing home reimbursement is perverse because it is focused on estimates of time required by various personnel to care for particular types of elders. The result is that the more an elder needs help with ADLs, exhibits behavioral problems, or requires nursing procedures, the more the institution is reimbursed. Dependent elders are thus more valuable, from a reimbursement standpoint, than more functional elders, especially when the more functional elder can act in opposition to or be noncompliant with institutional regimens. The result of these incentives is that 'enthusiasm for making residents less dependent is muted' (Kane and Kane 1990: 87). Time spent motivating and instructing elders is excluded from the calculations, a fact that has not escaped astute administrators. Because reimbursement is determined on the basis of the efficient provision of specific, discrete services and not on overall improvement in the quality of care or life of the elder, interactions become routinized. In effect, the entire atmosphere of the nursing home becomes regimented and mechanized. In part, this is understandable given the production mentality of the medical model that strongly influences the provision of care for elders. It is small consolation that things are not much better with home care. The payment system reimburses only those providers who have been formally certified by regulatory agencies. Hence, elders are basically prevented from recruiting their own help. A defender of negative freedom might, of course, object that elders are not forced to forego hiring help of their own choosing, provided, of course, that they can pay for it. When ability to pay is limited, reliance on social services effectively constrains choice. This does seem to violate the positive requirements of autonomy. If enhancement or preservation of autonomy is a goal of long-term care, then the restriction of choice by regulation is a subject deserving careful analysis.

Medicare does not provide reimbursement for services needed to maintain independent functioning such as transportation away from the nursing home. Institutionalized elders are thus unable to freely visit families, pursue their own chosen activities, or develop their own schedules, whenever their incapacities restrict their movements. Effectively, they are incarcerated in the institutions in which they live. Empirical work has shown striking dissonance between the preferences expressed by the elders and those acknowledged by staff. Elders rate trips out of the facility and the use of the telephone as very important, whereas staff most often regard organized nursing home activities such as bingo or arts and crafts as most important and least often think that using the telephone was important at all (Kane et al. 1990: 70).

One conclusion that could be drawn from these observations is that nursing homes simply need reform. Guided by the ideal of autonomy as independence, one can insist that institutionalized elders need to be set free, liberated. Liberation is unquestionably an appropriate implication of a concern for autonomy in long-term care, but one should scrupulously inquire into the actual conditions requisite for liberation. For colonial states, liberation is a justifiable political goal, but achieving that goal does not guarantee the economic sufficiency necessary for true state sovereignty. Analogously, liberation for elders in nursing homes is a far too simplistic proposal if it follows the political tack of aiming for independence alone. Similarly, reforms that focus on the institutional structure of nursing homes or on specific problems without an adequate understanding of the framework supporting positive views of autonomy are likely to prove ineffectual. Such a framework is also needed to counter latent generalizations about what it is to be old in our society. These generalizations form a sedimentary layer that impedes progress. This layer needs excavation and evaluation. Attitudes and beliefs that underlie explanations of the behavior of elders such as 'that's the way they are when they're old' (Shield 1988: 16) involve treating elders abstractly, as members of a category rather than as individuals. In a sense, elders seldom are seen as *us*, but as somehow fundamentally different and alien. Regarding elders as other is an example of a wider phenomenon of treating as alien things that constitute a fundamental threat to our own sense of self or well-being (Gilman 1988). This behavior can be confronted not by insisting that autonomy be respected, but by probing further into the seminal meanings of long-term care that shape our understanding of autonomy's place therein.

One concept central in long-term care that functions in nursing homes in particular is that of the therapeutic relationship. Although there is some disagreement over whether a social or medical approach is best in the management of particular cases or as a philosophy of long-term care, the overall model is therapeutic. The therapeutic model, however, contains powerful expectations like *following doctor's orders* that effectively shape, and some would say inhibit, the style and substance of interactions necessary for autonomy to thrive in long-term care. To appreciate the effect that this might have on autonomy, it is worthwhile considering the expectations generally associated with the concept of the therapeutic in contemporary society.

Therapeutic relationships

A *therapeutic relationship* is a relationship between an individual who suffers some defect, disability, or discomfort and a practitioner who possesses a specific technical skill or knowledge and who occupies a recognized social role. The primary goal of the relationship is to improve the well-being of the suffering individual as the result of action that is undertaken within the relationship. It is no wonder, then, that professional medical ethics is frequently described as an agency ethic (American College of Physicians 1984b: 266; Beauchamp and Childress 1983: 213; Daniels 1986: 1382; Fried 1978: 243; Pellegrino and Thomasma 1981: 275), that is, an ethic in which the practitioner is obligated to function as the agent of the patient, acting in the patient's best interest as determined by professional judgment. Although this ethic has often been tarred with the brush of paternalism, there are important considerations that support carefully distinguishing paternalism and beneficence as discussed in Chapter 2. For present purposes, it is important to note that the definition of well-being pursued and the judgments made regarding the presenting problem (the defect, deficiency, or disability) are interrelated in complex ways that require reference to the specific practice in which the therapeutic relationship is a constituent part (Agich 1983b).

Therapeutic relationships exhibit three general interdependent features: a particular structure and style of interaction, a particular intention to improve or contribute to the well-being of an individual (as well as a particular definition or understanding of what constitutes sickness and well-being), and a particular set of techniques or skills that are possessed and exercised by the practitioner that can broadly be referred to as therapeutic. It is thus assumed or required that possession of expert knowledge, skill, or technique is an essential feature of being a practitioner. As a corollary, practitioners acquire a special power over patients, a power that naturally gives rise to concerns about paternalism.

The definition just offered defines the essential features of therapeutic relationships in general. Individual kinds of therapeutic relationships exhibit these features in a variety of ways. By focusing on the kinds of skill, techniques, or interactions that are possible and the correlative definitions of the well-being sought, one can develop a taxonomy of therapeutic relationships. Historically, not only medicine and health care, but also philosophy, religion, and art were seen as therapeutic. In Western societies, the dominant understanding of the therapeutic is based on the sick role as represented in acute care medicine. This model assumes an asymmetrical relationship between the sick person and therapeutic agencies.

The *sick role* has three primary elements: first, the acceptance by both self and others that being ill is not the sick person's fault and that she should be seen more as a victim of forces beyond her control; second, there is a claimed exemption from usual daily expectations and obligations; and third, if the illness is sufficiently severe, then the sick person will seek help from a health care provider (Parsons 1975: 262). The sick role concept captures the predominant social model of illness in our society. To understand the way that the sick role influences our thinking about autonomy in long-term care requires reflecting on how therapeutic relationships are modeled in the practice of medicine.

The therapeutic practice constitutes a backdrop that defines the nature of well-being and shapes judgments about disability or disease. The practice thus includes background beliefs and values that shape the individual actions undertaken in the name of therapy. This point is important. Chapter 4 develops the idea that identification with beliefs, choices, and values that are truly one's own logically precedes freedom and is the core element in autonomy of persons. If this argument is sound, then the fact that the experience and perception of individuals in long-term care fail to correspond with those of long-term caregivers certainly creates conflicts that activate concern for autonomy as negative freedom. Autonomy is, however, also threatened at the more basic level of underlying belief and value. Alienation of individual elders from the socially defined sick role and the meanings associated with disease diagnosis is thus not only possible, but perhaps inevitable. This fact poses important ethical questions. Human existence is essentially social, yet the autonomy of persons involves identifications that can creatively depart from social norms or expectations. Tensions, if not contradictions, are therefore unavoidable. An approach that can constructively deal with these differences not only as practical problems to be resolved, but also as involving basic questions of virtue, value, and character, is sorely needed (May 1986).

Philip Rieff's discussion of the striking difference between what he termed *classical* (or traditional) and *modern* views of therapy (1966) is helpful in making this point. Modern views of therapy primarily concern *what cures*. Classical views were concerned with *who cures*. On the classical view, it was ultimately the community that cured, because the function of the classical therapist was to reintegrate the patient into the symbol system of the community by means of specialized techniques sanctioned by the community, for example ritual, dialectical, magical, or rational techniques. As Rieff put it:

All such efforts to reintegrate the subject into the community symbol system may be categorized as 'commitment therapies.' Behind shaman and priest, philosopher and physician stems the great community as the ultimate corrective of personal disorders. (1966: 68–9)

Modern views of therapy, however, function where the community itself is disordered and not able to supply a system capable of symbolic integration. As a result, the therapeutic capacity of the community is lost or compromised; instead, it is transferred to a specialized group of individuals who treat patients as individuals, and not as representatives of the community. An implication of this changed view of therapy is that caregiving, too, is transformed from an activity that is readily available and disseminated within the community to an activity that is separate and apart from everyday life and surrounded by a special professional aura. Therapy thus becomes something pursued and achieved only in special professional relationships. To be sure, shamans certainly enjoyed a special aura, yet their function was open to the community in that their actions expressed deeply held and widely shared beliefs and values. Mystery, of course, always surrounds a good deal of modern as well as classical therapeutic proceedings, but in classical therapy it is attached to the community and the sick individual by a shared worldview in which the nature and meaning of sickness are continuous with everyday experience. In the modern world that is not the case.

Despite cultural faith in scientific progress, the central meanings of the biomedical and clinical sciences are hardly continuous with everyday experience and structures of explanation. One important result is that there is dissonance between patient and physician understandings of illness. This dislocation or separation creates a different kind of mystery from that of the classical world and a different kind of power for the modern health professional when compared with traditional healers. In the modern world the sick individual is, by virtue of the sickness, literally transformed into a patient and is thus different from others, especially the physician, whose agency is seen as fully intact. Patients are supposed to be passive and are simply expected to take their medicine; it is not necessary that the patient's view of illness accord with the physician's understanding. The main requirement is compliance with doctor's orders, and that is mostly a matter of undergoing the physician's interventions, not a matter of the patient's personal belief.

The power of modern medicine thus rests on its causal efficaciousness without the need for a concordance of belief between healer and patient. As a result, in the modern concept of the therapeutic, truth is displaced as a value and the patient's autonomous agency is marginalized. The patient does not need to believe, understand, or know, because modern medicine operates outside the sphere of communal or personal validation, relying instead on scientific knowledge to treat disease. The modern concept of the therapeutic thus has little need for widespread social understanding or support, relying instead on a narrower and specialized scientific standard of truth. Specialized scientific knowledge rather than a communal system of belief is pivotal. Of course, one might object that this scientific standard of truth is itself socially accepted. That is certainly true, but the acceptance is predicated on a global and mostly blind faith in scientific progress and technology rather than on an understanding of even key scientific concepts and acceptance of scientific beliefs. The acceptance of science is thus predicated less on the meaningful way that it explains common social experience than on its power as technology (Agich 1981). There exists a striking gap between scientific and everyday modes of explanation that permeates the modern view of therapy as well.

Since the therapeutic has become appropriated as a concept of specialized professional knowledge, the sick person is conceived to lack the personal resources to help herself. On this view, then, autonomy is by definition waived or compromised by illness. The sick individual becomes fully a patient and so ceases to be an agent (MacIntyre 1977). In this regard it is enlightening to note that informed consent is a uniquely modern development. Informed consent requires disclosure of information regarding the treatment proposed, its risks and benefits, as well as the alternative treatments available to patients in order to allow them to accept (or reject) the treatment based on their personal preferences and values. Informed consent reflects not only the prominence of individual self-determination in the modern world; it functions precisely in a social context in which solidarity or shared commitment to a belief system is rare. To be a therapist of individuals, who are independent and isolated from a wider community of meaning, thus requires that the therapist be similarly severed or disconnected from the community at large. The predictable result is that not binding sentiment, but critical detachment becomes the attitude presumed to be conducive to a sense of well-being in the modern view (MacIntyre 1981: 29; cf. Koch 1971).

While concepts of health and disease may be based on consensus regarding values and beliefs, cure or successful therapy may not be achievable simply by the power of consensus or public opinion. There are obvious limits to the power of consensus to correct or ameliorate serious defects, disabilities, or discomforts. One cannot rationally expect that even widely shared beliefs will prevent or cure disease or correct disabilities or discomforts, because the relation of beliefs to effective action is not logical, but empirical. Widespread or strong belief in an intervention alone does not assure the effectiveness of the intervention. This point is true enough, but perhaps its usefulness is limited. If informed consent is important, then patient beliefs and values, even regarding what is (wrongly thought to be) therapeutically efficacious, should be taken into account by health care providers. Interestingly, the importance of patient beliefs and values has been identified by Lidz, Appelbaum, and Meisel (1988) as one of the phases of a process (in contrast to a disclosure) model of informed consent, and by Pankratz and Kofoed (1988) as a recommendation for assessing and treating 'geezers,' whose own values are the key to establishing an effective therapeutic relationship. That social role and causal effectiveness can be separated is shown by the fact that people may be able to heal or actually suffer independently of the opinion of their society (Neu 1975: 112). In long-term care, where the scientific understanding of disease process is more limited than for many acute illnesses and health professionals are singularly incapable of achieving a cure, even more space for patient autonomy should be provided.

The distinction between modern and classical views of therapy and the therapeutic relationship would be misleading if it were taken either to indicate that medicine and, particularly, the modern physician–patient relationship are not supported by social consensus or that therapeutic power is simply a direct result of social consensus. Historical evidence seems to contradict both of these conclusions. The way that acute care medicine provides the dominant model for long-term care, however, introduces assumptions that support an individualistic view of therapy and a concept of the causal effectiveness of therapeutic interventions that are radically different from the classical view described by Rieff. The implications of this distinction can be made clear by focusing on the nature of illness and disease in our society.

Concepts of illness and disease

In modern medicine, illness or disease is not defined positively, but privatively in terms of an inability to exercise rational free agency (Engelhardt 1976). This may be due either to the absence of a strong social consensus regarding a positive definition of well-being or to recognition of the empirical and fallible character of diagnosis itself. Whatever its cause, defining well-being or health negatively in terms of disease categories appears to be the dominant view in contemporary medicine. Thus, those conditions or states of affairs that reduce or restrict rational free action tend to count as diseases and those states that augment rational free action count as health (Engelhardt 1976).

One implication of this view is that concepts of health and disease are plastic or malleable. Because rational free agency and choice are abstract concepts that can express any number of value commitments, what counts as a disease in contemporary medicine largely depends on what types of suffering human beings as finite rational agents are willing to accept and on the kind of lives they wish to live. These judgments are not the product of idiosyncratic or individual preference alone. They reflect a general, social view predominant at certain historical periods regarding what supports or thwarts autonomy. Consensus is involved but the consensus concerns certain abstract or general values and norms whose specification is left to the practice of medicine as a historical and empirical enterprise. The availability of techniques for intervening in and altering the undesirable states or conditions that compromise autonomy figures importantly in defining what counts as a disease.

Since autonomy is understood in this model in a general and abstract fashion, virtually anything that restricts rational free agency tends to count as disease. As a consequence, aging itself has been regarded as a disease, as something disvalued, because it entails a restriction on rational free action (Caplan 1984; Engelhardt 1979). Acceptance of the so-called life-span paradigm regarding what growing old involves permeates mainstream bioethical work on aging. The life-span paradigm is at work in the literature concerned with the social justice problem of resource scarcity as the population ages and end-of-life decision making in the face of the perceived loss of personal autonomy and meaning associated with being old (Agich 2001).

Deep-seated attitudes and beliefs about growing old shape the view that not only do elders suffer from diseases that are shared with younger members of society, they also suffer from the pervasive disease of living a long life, namely, being old. Regarding being old as a kind of disease reflects and reinforces the idea that dependence is problematic. This idea grows out of the association of disease and autonomy in contemporary medicine. In particular, dependence due to disability or frailty that is not remediable as such constitutes a fundamental disvalue of those who are impaired. Even among the old, those who are more impaired or frail are subject to attitudes and behaviors that reflect revulsion, as occurs under the newer versions of the elderly mystique (Cohen 1988).

The impact of these ideas of disease on long-term care is significant. First, the dominant model of disease reinforces existing social values regarding the aversion for dependency. In most situations, medical treatment is a tolerated interference in our everyday lives only insofar as it aims at (and achieves) cure. Such a goal, however, is both inappropriate and cruel in long-term care. Because such expectations cannot be met, caregivers are discouraged from offering real care and instead accept the inevitability of dependence. It is no wonder, then, that long-term care focuses on bed and body work and the person who is the subject of such work is forgotten. It is as if the elder as an autonomous agent ceased to exist once it became clear that ideal independence could not be restored. Contemporary medicine does not provide a sufficient basis upon which to establish a truly therapeutic environment for the impaired or frail elders. Since it cannot cure the problems that underlie dependence, medicine reflects the same social disvaluation not only of the specific illnesses of elders, but their very existential status as old and frail.

Models of care

One difficulty that confronts discussion of the problem of autonomy in long-term care is that medical ethics, like medicine itself, is acute care and in-patient oriented. Typically, a patient is institutionalized for short periods of time for discrete problems: the majority of care is provided by cadres of health professionals, who usually have brief procedure-oriented or task-oriented encounters with the patient. Clinical decision making, too, typically has a short time horizon: the goal is improvement of biological status to the point that permits discharge. Discharge is usually predicated on removal from the unit, not necessarily discharge from the hospital. The goal of resuming normal activities or regaining a premorbid quality of experience and range of activities is hardly ever explicitly the main object of concern for health professionals even though these are typically the preoccupation for patient and family. Restoration of normal arterial blood gases, for example, is a primary goal for pulmonologists and nurses in pulmonary and intensive care units, but it is rare for these scores to be related in any meaningful way to the patient's future lifestyle except, and only until, they are normalized or therapeutic defeat acknowledged. The orientation is thus exceedingly short term, problem defined, and task dominated. Bureaucratic organization of the delivery of services further exacerbates the alienation of health professionals from the patient as a person.

Given the dominance of the acute care orientation in American medicine, it is not at all surprising that bioethical thinking has come to focus on the paradigm cases and problems that arise in acute care medical settings. This focus is usually marked by crisis and conflict. Ethics becomes relevant only when all else fails, because the basic orientation is on specific problems, procedures, and tasks. Given the structural features of the way health care is delivered, conflict is inevitable

Conflict arises under conditions of great stress and under circumstances that do afford sufficient opportunity to ameliorate disagreement. It is no wonder, then, that rights language has come to dominate medical ethics. Profoundly influenced by medical–legal developments, medical ethics has wholly adopted, and certainly adapted, concepts such as informed consent that had their origin in the malpractice arena (Faden and Beauchamp 1986). The consequence is that legalism is a dominant feature of medical ethics, which helps explain why medical ethics tends to focus on conflictual and dramatic problems and relies heavily on the language of rights instead of, for example, the language of responsibility (Agich 1982; Ladd 1978).

Conflict is also inevitable because of the fundamental orientation of acute medical care toward patient welfare as judged by the physician. Beneficence dominates this model. It is accepted because the disruption posed by sickness or illness is usually limited and reversible. The physician can arrive at relatively unambiguous determinations of patient need and reliable assessments of the risks and benefits associated with proposed or alternate therapies. Informed consent or, better still, informed choice involves presenting patients with an array of options that are discrete and readily understandable. The physician defines patient needs as well as the risks and benefits associated with treatment for the patient. In long-term care, however, the principle of beneficence is less powerful and so affords weaker basis for caregiver authority. This principle is less dominant because physicians are usually only remotely involved in long-term care and usually at some distance from day-to-day treatment. As a result, autonomy becomes not only more important, but also takes on positive features lacking in the acute care-based medical model that supports simple informed choice.

Elders who need long-term care suffer from chronic conditions that are not curable. Risks and benefits cannot be readily ascertained and, in any event, clearly involve elements that are not necessarily excluded by the much more diffuse model of long-term care. For example, the sick role concept underlying acute care assumes that the sick person will cooperate with health professionals to restore premorbid functioning, indeed, has the obligation to do so. Long-term care by definition precludes a return to premorbid, normal functioning, so personal or idiosyncratic considerations that would otherwise be trumped by the obligation to get well retain their validity. Long-term care needs also tend to involve multiple, overlapping physical, psychological, and social dimensions that cannot all be readily conceptualized, much less managed, in strict medical terms (Hofland 1988: 5).

Even for clear medical needs there is often greater uncertainty and a wider range of possible interventions. Because the goal cannot be cure, the diagnostic therapeutic certainty of the acute care model finds little to grip. Lacking the traction provided by the goal of curing as the main ingredient of patient welfare, patient preferences and values become far more important. In the acute care context, especially in hospitals, the foreign environment intimidates patients. In contrast, home care is delivered on the patient's own turf and institutional care occurs where the patient resides, so patient autonomy is in a more fertile environment. Despite these environmental differences, long-term care, especially nursing home care, seems to efface rather than enhance the residual autonomy of elders.

The nursing home mystique exerts a subtle and pervasive influence on thinking about long-term care. Largely because of the migration of the medical model into the nursing home, the emphasis is on medical or nursing care even though there seems to be little such care actually given. Typically, nursing homes are structured in form and circumstance very much like hospitals: physical arrangement of rooms, furniture, maintenance of records, distribution of medications, presence of a nursing station even though most care is provided by aides rather than trained nurses. These structural elements affect the everyday practice of caregiving in nursing homes; collectively, they convey powerful expectations about who the elder is and what is the elder's proper role. This is evident in the way that the medical condition of individuals who live in nursing homes tends to dominate much of the formal structure as well as day-to-day activity (Gubrium 1975; Lidz, Fischer, and Arnold 1990; Savishinsky 1991; Shield 1988). Elders are referred to by their medical condition, their unit or room number, or simply as 'that patient' (Lidz, Fischer, and Arnold 1990: 69–86). Elders seem no more differentiating about staff than members of staff are about elders. In their ethnographic study of autonomy in long-term care, Lidz, Fischer, and Arnold reported that despite considerable efforts at explanation, their female observer was sometimes called 'nurse' even though she wore street clothes and provided no nursing care. Patients seemed either unable or disinterested in making any distinctions between the different staff members who cared for them (1990: 69–70).

The history and sociology of nursing homes are part of a larger phenomenon, namely, the institutionalization of social deviants, such as criminals, indigents, the insane and orphans. Rothman (1971) convincingly argued that the trend toward institutionalization in the United States was mainly an attempt to deal with a wide range of problems, such as crime, poverty, and severe illness, that were seen for the first time as social in nature. Institutions were seen as serving both preventive and rehabilitative purposes, particularly in Jacksonian America, and were developed on the basis of principles and routine. Programs were designed to separate the aged chronically ill and disabled from those able to work, to allow each institution to impose a special routine on its particular population. This heritage of regimentation and social engineering is evident in nursing homes today. It is, however, mediated by the development of specific medical institutions like the acute care hospital that has exerted such a profound influence on the structure of American medicine and medical ethics and is supported by a payment system that rewards efficiency in the provision of specific services, but not necessarily care of elders as such (Kane and Kane 1990).

The federal regulation of nursing homes involves two major sets of regulatory requirements. One contains the requirements that facilities must meet to participate in Medicare and Medicaid (Code of Federal Regulations 1987a, 1987b). The second covers the enforcement process that the federal government and its agents, namely, the state survey agencies, must follow in inspecting nursing homes and approving or disapproving them for participation (Code of Federal Regulations 1987c). When this process began in 1965 with the creation of Medicare, long-term care facilities presented special problems because no regulatory model existed for either skilled or intermediate care facilities. The Joint Commission hospital or medical model did exist and that model was adapted to derive a new set of regulations for nursing homes (Morford 1988: 129).

Two concerns dominated these regulations: safety and adequacy of treatment services. Addressing physical safety was relatively straightforward. The facilities should be fire-safe and clean and staff should not abuse patients. These concerns are the so-called bricks and mortar requirements designed to improve patient safety in America's nursing homes. Adequacy of treatment and services, however, was not easily addressed. One should not think that successful surgery will occur in hospitals simply by mandating success in surgery, but one can try to promote that outcome, requiring surgeons to meet specific qualifications or follow appropriate procedures and policies. In nursing homes, the same principles were applied; detailed policies, procedures, and qualifications were promulgated in lieu of direct outcome measures (Morford 1988: 129). There is reason to believe that these standards are generally outcome insensitive. Whether that is true or not is a complicated question, but it does seem evident that these standards are not particularly sensitive to promoting or maintaining autonomy in nursing home residents (Kane and Kane 1990). In fact, the burdens of complying with the standards, such as meeting record-keeping requirements, divert scarce staff time and effort from other activities. The overriding problem is that the nursing home regulations impose a task-oriented medical model of care on what might be better thought of in other terms.

The concept of a practice

To explore the impact of acute care medicine on the understanding of autonomy in medical ethics, it is useful to reflect on the similarities and differences between acute care medicine and long-term care as practices by considering first the defining features of a practice. Two general features of practices are important (Flathman 1976, 1980). The first is the rule-governed character of practices. A practice can be defined as a set of ordered activities that is characterized by patterns of regularity. The term rule refers not only to the seeming objective regularities that may be observed in the behaviors of participants in a practice that are catalogued by social scientists, but also to the regularities and norms that define the practice for the participants and that the participants in the practice knowingly and intentionally follow. In this sense, rules are less like objective laws of nature providing explanatory frameworks than they are like rules of thumb or recipes for action that all social actors, including social scientists, employ in engaging in particular practices.

The rules of a practice include the specialized knowledge, skills-at-hand, and procedures that normatively define the status of individuals as practitioners or as participants in the practice in question. Following rules and knowing which rules to follow are features that define individuals as participants in a practice. This is not simply an abstract requirement, but reflects actual experience. Behaviors and organizational structures associated with nursing homes discussed above, such as taking vital signs, charting care activities performed for patients, and bureaucratic organization, reflect rules derived from hospital-based care. To function as a caregiver in a nursing home involves learning a wide range of rules that are task oriented, geared toward helping elders to complete basic ADLs.

The rules of a practice, however, are not free standing. They depend on a logically distinct but related set of values and beliefs that provide participants a basis for accepting and following rules. Rules guide conduct only where there is acceptance of ways of thinking and acting that have a wider significance and relevance than the particular rules. In other words, rules must make sense to the participants; they must afford a basis for meaningful social action. What constitutes meaningful social action is determined in part by reference to values and beliefs of the participants. It is these values and beliefs that provide the basis on which participants regard rules as valuable and as deserving of their observance. Logically, such an understanding cannot be part of the formulation of any given rule or set of rules, but is a separate feature that defines practices.

Long-term care differs strikingly from acute-oriented hospital-based care. Some long-term care, like hospital care, is residential, but the latter is usually temporary and a return to normal activities and home is typically a reasonable goal. Most long-term care, however, does not occur in institutions at all but in the elder's own home. This fact makes quite a significant difference. In the case of hospital care, the temporary nature of the hospital stay coupled with the patients' (and families') desire and belief in its therapeutic benefit underlie acceptance of the loss of autonomy that patients regularly endure in hospitals. For example, the lives of patients are regimented. Restrictions are placed on when and if routine personal care such as bathing or showering can be undertaken, when and what foods and liquids may be consumed, what visitors one might entertain, the times during which one must sleep or awaken, and there is the tacit expectation that medication be taken and other doctor's orders followed. Typically, these restrictions amount to a lot of things done to a patient who has surrendered independence at least for the duration of the hospital stay. These and myriad other restrictions on freedom seem to be tolerated because of the temporary nature of most hospital stays and the underlying belief that a therapeutic benefit will result. As discussed above, patients even accept therapeutic benefit on the basis of the physician's inherent authority in medical matters.

It is not clear that such assumptions make any sense or are widely accepted in long-term care, certainly not in home-based care. There appears to be a widespread belief, perhaps reflective of a deep fear, that long-term care is permanent, to be interrupted only by acute episodes of illness that require hospitalization or, finally, by death. Once commenced, the process will inexorably wind down with ever-decreasing satisfaction and self-worth. The sense of independent agency or self-determination that is temporarily ceded in hospital care is thought to be lost or permanently foregone once institutional long-term care begins. This occurs even though the events that precipitate nursing home care are not necessarily parallel to acute illness. Typically, the illnesses and disabilities bringing individuals into long-term care are chronic and usually irremediable. Since cure is out of the question, it is perversely paradoxical that medical ways of thinking should prevail.

A plausible general view is that any practice should reveal its underlying beliefs and values, which justify or make sense of the rules guiding the participants in the practice in question, if only they are carefully examined. Judging from the ethnographic literature, however, the practice of long-term care, at least in nursing homes, presents a puzzling and paradoxical picture. The dominant influence of the medical model is pervasively insinuated into long-term care despite the fact that the underlying values and beliefs are widely recognized as inappropriate. A fundamental contradiction exists in this important institution of long-term care that the ethnographic work on nursing homes elaborately reveals. Fortunately, despite their cultural and social importance, nursing homes do not exhaust the full practice of long-term care.

Hospital and nursing home care occurs in places that are alien and intimidating to most patients. The situation is quite different when care occurs in an elder's own home. An elder, with few exceptions, is typically on native ground. Caregivers are for the most part family members. Unlike nursing homes (and hospitals) where the problem is how to instill caring into health professionals, the problem in home care is how to enable those who care for the patient to acquire the skills requisite for adequate care. Home health aides and homemakers who provide necessary personal care and homemaking services can also spend significant time with the disabled elder, but health care professionals such as nurses and physicians are only episodically involved, and certainly not on a daily basis. For the most part, the family bears the burden of caring for the disabled elder. Most elders want to remain in their familiar surroundings and receive care from those they know and love (Young 1990).

In light of these patterns of long-term caregiving, it is not at all safe to assume that therapeutic relationships can or should be conceptualized along the lines of the medical model. Long-term care is in reality a diffuse set of phenomena ranging from various formal and informal in-home help services, professional home nursing care to institutional skilled nursing and medical care. Long-term care is an extended family of practices rather than a single practice. Due to the dominance of the medical model in nursing homes, nursing homes set the paradigm for thinking about long-term care. There certainly seems to be much better evidence regarding institutional long-term care than home care. This is so because nursing homes are public institutions, whereas care provided at home by family or friends is private and, in an important sense, invisible to social scientists. Formal home care services are a recent development that is also receiving attention for its impact on the autonomy of elders (Pignatello, Taylor, and Young 1989; Young 1990; Young and Pelaez 1990). Some features of home care are uncontroversial and highly relevant to the question of autonomy in long-term care.

Home care

Families care for more elders than are cared for in institutions. The single largest group of caregivers is elders themselves, mostly spouses. Chronic care, in which day-to-day supervision or nursing is needed, seems to be the special province of family members. Elders seem to prefer family care to other forms of support. The evidence suggests that the norm of filial responsibility, despite its problems, enjoys significant compliance (Christiansen 1983: 27–8). Honoring these responsibilities, however, can be onerous. Even corporate America has become aware that its employees have family caregiving responsibilities that affect the workplace. Elder care has been described as an emerging employee benefit of the 1990s (Azarnoff and Scharach 1988).

For the most part, women are in the middle of the dependent care contin-uum. They have responsibilities for parents or sometimes for grandparents on one side and their own children on the other. No doubt this introduces sig-nificant stresses. One observer has captured the intergenerational dimension of balancing responsibilities to children with responsibilities to elder parents with the phrase *the sandwich generation* (Brody 1985). With the growth in the elderly population, it is no wonder that political programs have spurred the development of home health from a cottage industry into a formal sector of health care. These developments have prompted reflection on the unique ques-tion of autonomy in home care settings (Dubler 1990; Kapp 1990; Pignatello, Taylor, and Young 1989; Sabatino 1990a; Young 1990).

Because home care includes various homemaking, social, as well as medical or nursing services, it hardly matches the medical model described earlier.

The medical model defines the sick person's needs in medical terms for management by a professional in a professionalized setting. The sick person is expected to cooperate with therapy and to adapt to all its inconveniences with the goal of returning to normal functioning. Care for chronic conditions of old age rendered in the home, however, does not meet these basic conditions. Not only is cure impossible by definition, the mode of treatment frequently consists of services that in large part aim at fulfilling the elder's daily living needs. Many are basic housekeeping or help functions, not specific nursing or medical services. In this context, there is no overriding authority comparable to that wielded by the physician in the medical model, understandably so because many elements of home care are relatively nonmedical.

Informed consent that operationalizes the principle of autonomy in the medical care model is not of central import in the home care setting because its foils, physician authority and physician-determined beneficence, are not readily apparent either. The elder is thus in a far better position to express her own values and beliefs and to maintain independent decision making. A largely ignored concern, though, is the implicit decisions made by spouse and children regarding various aspects of home care. This need not be a usurpation of the dependent elder's autonomy. Even when the family makes most of the key caregiving decisions, these still could be made with the approval of the dependent elder who willingly places herself in the hands of loved ones. What seems called for is an alternative to both the individual patient rights model and the virtuous (beneficent) practitioner model, a complementary alternative that Harry R. Moody termed a 'communicative ethic based on deliberation and negotiation' (1988: 69). Such a model would have to incorporate the responsibilities of the elder to reach accommodation with family caregivers (Dubler 1990). Indeed, the concern for abuse and exploitation in the home care setting, though certainly present in some cases, needs to be directed as much to caregivers as to elders because the balance of power frequently favors the elder. This fact alone is reason why philosophers should pay attention to home care.

Reciprocity in the home requires that the concept of negative freedom should be augmented by the use of more positive concepts that amplify the virtues and responsibilities of elders (Jameton 1988; May 1986). Responsibilities of elders constitute a significant, yet insufficiently recognized, aspect of autonomy. They comprise a part and define the limiting edge of autonomy. It is reported that patients often assume responsibilities in health care settings and that caregivers attribute responsibilities to them (Kelly and May 1982; Tagliaczzo and Mauksch 1979). If such behavior occurs to any significant degree, it prompts questions regarding its function in defining the social world of elders in long-term care. Responsibility implies a relationship with others, a relationship that is, at least implicitly, reciprocal. Responsibility relationships are not static but dynamic, changing as circumstances and capacities alter;

ultimately, how one carries out one's responsibilities contributes centrally to defining the kind of person one is.

Andrew Jameton (1988) pointed out that responsibilities in long-term care are complex. These responsibilities include at least the following: responsibility for performing specific mundane tasks like pushing other patients confined to wheelchairs, sewing for others, assisting in fixing beds or meals; responsibilities to caregivers such as expressing gratitude toward caregivers, complaining appropriately and understandingly to caregivers; basic responsibilities not to hit, insult, or otherwise abuse caregivers; responsibilities to observe or not violate institutional rules or the customs and daily routines in the home of a child caregiver; responsibilities to other patients and residents; personal responsibilities regarding self-care and grooming; and responsibilities to others outside the home or institution, for instance maintaining contacts with relatives or observing their birthdays or significant life events. Even elders with limited physical abilities can assume some of these responsibilities, though, like all responsibilities, these naturally conform to changes in capacity and circumstance and in large part reflect who an elder is and what are her defining beliefs and values as a person. An elder's failure to assume these kinds of responsibilities can attest to her isolation from a sense of family or social community and a deficient sense of personal worth as a moral agent.

If frail or incapacitated elders appear powerless, they can be empowered precisely by acknowledging them as responsible persons. Taking elders seriously as members of the moral community of persons entails understanding their obligations and responsibilities as well as respecting their rights. Failure to criticize elders may subtly remove them from the realm of persons; unlike very young children who are not usually held accountable for all their actions, elders are morally mature. To respect elders as moral agents, then, requires that we acknowledge and support the virtues and character traits appropriate to being old. Virtues involve not only the habits that allow us effectively to exercise our agency in the world, but comprise the strengths that grow out of adversities and sustain us through them (May 1986: 50).

William F. May (1986) complained that academics frequently think of themselves as critics of the arrogance of caregivers, but that they, too, contribute also to the power imbalance by concentrating exclusively on the ethics of caregivers and neglecting the ethics of care receivers. Ethics cannot adequately respect or enhance the moral being of elders in long-term care if it simply clears out a zone of indeterminate liberty for them while remaining indifferent to its particular uses. A liberty merely patronized is a moral being denied. Respect for the elder as person demands more than giving him berth, licensing him to do, say, or be whatever he pleases. Respect must include an additional moral give-and-take, a process of mutual deliberation, judgment, and criticism, and an occasional accounting for one another's views and deeds (May 1986: 48).

Taking the autonomy of elders seriously, then, involves exploring the kinds of moral bearing that old age requires. This is equally an issue in nursing homes as in home care, but home care presents unique complications owing to the power that elders maintains residing on their own turf and to the submerged dynamics in family relationships that invariably complicate matters. A new complication in home care is the introduction of professional caregivers of various sorts into the home, bringing with them alien (to the particular home or household) models of care and routines rife with strife.

The professionalization of home health care services under Medicare has had enormous impact on the development of home care. Medicare, the only wide-based, nonmeans-tested entitlement for home care, requires that agencies providing home care be certified and licensed. Individuals are virtually precluded from qualifying as a licensed provider. Medicare takes the most severe position of all, requiring that the client be homebound to qualify for home health care. Often a case manager is introduced and serves as an assessor who has final authority to decide what services are to be given, how often, and under what circumstances (Kane 1995; Wetle 1995). Elders, of course, have rights of refusal, but such rights are extremely costly for frail elders to exercise. The costs associated with such a refusal are not only individual but also social. Some kinds of care cannot be refused or are more difficult to refuse because of the way they are proffered.

Some caregiving involves special social relationships. Attached to these special relationships are sets of social expectations and obligations that importantly influence and structure individual behavior. In our society caregiving relationships such as parenting, teaching, or doctoring carry rather strong normative beliefs and values that influence the kind and range of options that individuals typically envision. The injection of the medical model into home care, even if still limited by many factors, is a cause for concern that merits research. For one thing, it introduces standards of care that if not tempered with judgment can fracture family relationships over technical issues of care when the emotional support and affective comfort provided to the frail elder by spouse or children outweigh any medical benefit that specialized professional help or institutionalization could ever bring.

Until the passage of the 1987 Budget Reconciliation Act, there were no specific client rights defined for home care services. By 1989 only 15 states had developed specific client rights articulated in statute or regulation. The Commission on Legal Problems of The Elderly of the American Bar Association (ABA) examined the effectiveness of these 'bills of rights' to enhance or at least prevent diminution of the autonomy of elders in long-term care (Sabatino 1989, 1990b). Virtually all the rights delineated in the statutes or regulations fall into one of five categories: informational rights (e.g., to be informed regarding services available by the agency, charges for services, one's medical condition, name, and method of contacting the provider's supervisor, and the affiliation of the agency with any organizations from whom or to whom referrals are made), participation and control rights (including participation in care planning, consent to or refusal of treatment, participation in evaluation of care, and access to one's clinical records), general civil rights and protections (to be treated with consideration, respect, and dignity, to be free from discrimination or from physical, psychological, or chemical abuse, to respect privacy and confidentiality of records and other information), remedial rights (such as to complain without fear of reprisals, to be told how to complain to the provider agency or state and local authorities), or quality rights (rights to safe and professional care, continuity of or timely care, or to be served by trained and competent personnel) (Sabatino 1990a: 22).

In reflecting on the two surveys of home care patient rights conducted by the ABA's Commission on Legal Problems of The Elderly, Charles P. Sabatino questioned whether rights language is at all appropriate to convey the positive expectations that the regulations intend. He noted that as the research proceeded, it became clear that the means of communicating with patients about their substantial legal rights, when expressed in rights language, deviated from the way elders really thought of home care providers. Rights language sounded to most elders adversarial and therefore posed a problem for elders who generally believed their caregivers were not even potentially their adversaries. When rights issues were reiterated in terms of expectations about home care, however, clients were more readily able and willing to respond. This was not simply a semantic distinction, but indicated fundamentally different ways of thinking about the nature of the relationship that the home care provider has with the elder that poses interesting questions concerning education of elders regarding their legal entitlements (Sabatino 1990a: 23–4).

These findings reinforce the point expressed earlier regarding the need for alternative way to conceptualize respecting the disabled or frail elder in the home. The language of rights is just too strident and distracting in the intimate space of the home. Notions of filial responsibility and accountability seem far more promising. An ethics of home care, unlike medical ethics or nursing home ethics, cannot comfortably rely on advocacy for the elder. The elder at home is, after all, not always powerless. The ethic of strangers that a patient rights approach supports seems singularly misplaced in the home setting. Instead, an ethic of intimates is sorely needed.

Summary

The question of autonomy in long-term care is entangled in the mythology surrounding aging and long-term care in our society. Specific treatment of autonomy in long-term care has to start with the recognition of the contextual meaning of the specific care functions involved. Long-term care is a rather diffuse set of caregiving activities ranging from housekeeping help in the home to skilled nursing home care. If to be autonomous does not mean absolute independence, but involves a situated or contextual freedom, then those social institutions and relationships comprising long-term care have to be examined in some detail in order to identify practices that enhance or thwart autonomy. This includes how decision making actually occurs, the actual daily routines and styles of caregiving, and the environmental factors that enhance or thwart autonomy.

It is important to realize that respect for autonomy cannot mean that caregivers are absolutely precluded from influencing the decisions of elders. To be exposed to influence is not to be enslaved. In fact, we need to acknowledge that the relationship between the receiver of care and the caregiver is far more complicated, especially in long-term care, than the standard medical model implies. As discussed earlier, the paradigm assumes that the health professional is in a position of power and authority over the patient. Hence, the patient must be protected from this power and authority. In some long-term care settings, especially when care is provided by family or in the patient's home or when the elder is cognitively and decisional competent and cared for in a nursing home by underpaid and overworked staff, the situation is likely to be reversed, that is, the elder retains power and some measure of independence. This is why the elder's responsibilities as an autonomous moral agent have to be given equal weight to any claim about the value of noninterference for the elder.

Concern for these matters prompted me to argue for an alternative framework, an alternative strategy for approaching the question of autonomy in long-term care (Agich 1990c). The next two chapters carry out this analysis in two ways. Chapter 4 deals with the more typical concern of autonomy as choice and defends a view that respecting autonomy as choice requires careful attention to the values and beliefs of the individuals involved. I argue that identification is more fundamental than free choice in understanding actual autonomy. Chapter 5 presses this analysis further by laying out a phenomenological account of some of the structural features of the world of everyday life that influence what it actually means to be an autonomous agent.

4

Actual autonomy

A significant problem with most liberal-inspired accounts of autonomy is the inadequacy of the underlying political model, namely, state sovereignty, for understanding personal autonomy. On the political model, the person is understood by analogy with an ideally autonomous political unit that is characterized by independence from the laws and governance of other states. To be autonomous in this sense is to be sovereign within a specific political domain. Influenced by this idea, many naturally think of the autonomy of the individual as analogously involving independence from the authority of others (state, institutions, or other individuals). Autonomy is thus defined privately as negative freedom in terms of that absence of coercion or dependence (Berlin 1969: 122; Young 1986: 3). This view of autonomy as negative freedom, though dominant, presents an intractable problem for long-term care only if it proves impossible to develop a complementary positive account that can accommodate the concrete character of autonomous action under conditions of dependence.

Most commentators agree that autonomy is a richly ambiguous and multi-textured concept that refers to a wide range of positively regarded attributes. This wide range of usage suggests that it is unlikely that any essential definition could unify these various usages (Dworkin 1988: 6). The central concepts involved in discussions of autonomy, such as consent, paternalism, or respect for persons, have such widely varying meanings partly because of their employment in different ethical theories (O'Neill 1984: 173). These different articulations of such fundamental concepts have important implications for assessing autonomy in long-term care. This diversity of usage might frustrate our inquiry were it not possible to order this theoretical morass. Onora O'Neill (1984) has developed a taxonomy of ethical theories that helpfully categorizes the main alternatives: result-oriented ethics; action-oriented ethics that takes an abstract view of autonomy, cognition, and volition; and action-oriented ethics that considers the determinate cognitive and volitional capacities and incapacities of particular individuals at particular times. The phrase *respect for autonomy* has very different meanings and implications in each of these types of theories.

Result-oriented theories

Most consequentialist or result-oriented ethics do not take patient autonomy to be a fundamental constraint on medical practice. For example, utilitarian thinking regards the production of welfare or well-being as the criterion of right action. Only when respect for patient autonomy maximizes welfare is it required. In this view, paternalistic abridgment of autonomy is not morally wrong in itself, but is wrong only when paternalistic action fails to achieve welfare or utility maximization. Commentators often overlook this point, because of John Stuart Mill's (1978) influential discussion of autonomy and paternalism in *On Liberty*. Mill offered such an eloquent defense of liberty that proponents of autonomy overlook that his defense is not really an argument in favor of autonomy as a basic ethical principle. Mill actually argued that each person is the judge of his or her own happiness and that the autonomous pursuit of one's goals is itself a major source of happiness; therefore, happiness seldom could be maximized by actions that thwarted or disregarded another's goals. The gist of the standard interpretation of Mill's utilitarian defense of autonomy is that we cannot make people better off, that is, promote their happiness, if individual autonomy is restricted. This interpretation of Mill is commonplace, though not without controversy, because there are features of Mill's treatment of liberty that cannot be readily squared with this interpretation. James Bogan and Daniel Farrell (1978), for example, argued that when Mill identifies happiness as the unique intrinsically desirable end, he does not necessarily mean a subjective state attained when desires are satisfied; rather he means something much broader, namely, the composite of ends that include health, liberty, virtue, and so forth. For this reason, he can regard autonomy as desirable for its own sake, even if it does not produce the subject state for which it was originally desired. On this interpretation, then, Mill's position is rather close to the view that autonomy is intrinsically desirable. Nevertheless, for the sake of argument we shall follow O'Neill's characterization of Mill's account as a primary example of a result-oriented theory.

The foundation of the utilitarian complaint against paternalists is that they *miscalculate* rather than pursue welfare for another and thereby *violate autonomy*. The central place that Mill assigned to autonomy in *On Liberty* is rather anomalous given his overall result-oriented ethical theory (Dworkin 1983). The impression that autonomy is primary in this account is thus misleading, because consequences are primary for Mill (and utilitarians), not free action. Apparently, because Mill believed that respecting autonomy leads to the consequences desired, namely, maximization of welfare, autonomy – or, more accurately, liberty – is supported as a basic social value.

Utilitarian theory requires that one calculate the expected utility or welfare based on empirical evidence and act on the results of such calculations. This is an important, yet often conveniently overlooked, feature of utilitarian thought. In empirical terms, Mill's claim that respecting liberty or individual free choice will lead to a maximization of welfare or utility may be false. For example, people may be happier under beneficent policies even when these reduce the scope of autonomous action. It would be an exaggeration to say that the matter can be settled by appeal to empirical evidence. It is exceedingly difficult to assess whether individuals actually do prize autonomy above happiness or welfare to the degree that Mill (along with many other philosophers) assumed. Instead, many individuals seem to want relief from difficult decisions associated with autonomy. Choosing can sometimes be burdensome. This seems to be the case with some types of medical decision making and may help explain why patients often ask their physicians 'What would you do?'. If this is true, then the utilitarian defense of autonomy against paternalism fails or is seriously weakened. If this line of interpretation is correct, what conclusions follow?

One way to interpret Mill's argument is as a defense of political liberty or noninterference and not autonomy of persons as an ethical value. As such, it is possible that *On Liberty* contains two distinctive, but not necessarily consistent, lines of argument: a utilitarian, result-oriented argument and a nonconsequentialist argument asserting that autonomy is a fundamental and irreducible condition of being a moral agent. O'Neill adopts the former interpretation. Even on this interpretation, Mill's account is still compatible with our earlier defense of the liberal theory of political autonomy. As an argument regarding the public, and hence political, merit of liberty, Mill's defense of liberty is important, even if the theoretical grounds of the defense are not immune from exegetical dispute. For present purposes, it is sufficient to note that the enthusiasm with which anti-paternalism is touted as a corollary of autonomy in medical ethics appears paradoxical, if it is true that one of the core anti-paternalist texts is not itself a defense of autonomy as a fundamental value, but only as an instrument for social welfare.

Taking Mill's treatment of autonomy in *On Liberty* as an illustration of result-oriented theories, these theories characteristically treat autonomy as a justified ethical value not in its own terms, but in terms of other, more fundamental considerations. The widespread acceptance of patient autonomy (and patient rights) as a central principle of medical ethics is supported by the way that appeals to patient autonomy and rights can help to curb the power and pretensions of health care providers and institutions rather than by a systematic analysis and justification of autonomy as a fundamental value in health care.

Action-oriented theories

Autonomy as an ethical concept can have a truly central place only in a different kind of ethical framework. An ethical theory that focuses on action rather than consequences is required to fully appreciate the fundamental preconditions of human agency. Autonomy is a central presupposition of agency; therefore, action-centered ethics must take the autonomy of agents to be a basic, rather than, as in utilitarian theory, a derivative ethical concern. This is true no matter how any particular action-centered theory defines the fundamental ethical category. Regardless of whether human rights, human worth, personhood, or principles of obligation constitute the basic ethical category, autonomy is involved. Following Kant, autonomy is commonly expressed as an obligation not to use other persons as means merely, but to respect them or treat them as ends in themselves. One main implication of this view in medical ethics is the doctrine of informed consent that imposes an obligation on health professionals to disclose information about risks, benefits, and alternatives of any proposed treatment and to avoid coercion or manipulation in medical decision making.

O'Neill (1984: 174), however, pointed out that action-oriented theories are quite diverse. Some view autonomy in abstract or formal terms, for example as a transcendental precondition for the possibility of morality (Kant); others see autonomy as a concrete existential condition of being a person or moral agent in the world. The distinction between abstract action-oriented and actual action-oriented theories is crucial for long-term care (Agich 1990c). Like result-oriented ethical theories, both types of action-oriented ethical theories have to face empirical difficulties and practical limitations that are especially pertinent in long-term care. Some individuals in long-term care clearly lack cognitive and volitional capacities that would warrant thinking of them as nonautonomous. Confronted by limited capacities, it is not practically useful to offer an analysis predicated on idealized examples that avoid the fundamental question posed in the concrete case. If autonomous action is ruled out in a broad range of long-term care cases, because the elders lack full cognitive and volitional capacity, then what is the ground for insisting on respecting or supporting their autonomy?

This question is central to the present study of the place of autonomy in long-term care. Transcribing the concrete case to a theoretical or idealized plane only bypasses the question. This question is also important for medical ethics generally, since patients routinely exhibit reduced cognitive and volitional capacities as the result of disease or psychological defenses. Illness represents a fundamental compromise or ontological assault on the basic existential conditions necessary for action in the world (Pellegrino and Thomasma 1981: 207–8). Saying this, of course, does not deny that many patients do have the capacity for agency. For these patients, an agency-centered or action-oriented ethics would be obviously relevant. For the problematic cases, however, only agent-centered moral theories that accurately assess the realities of human autonomy and human personhood will prove relevant (O'Neill 1984). Mainline interpretations of agent-centered ethics, however, are not helpful precisely because they tend to rely on an abstract and inaccurate view of autonomy.

The abstract view of autonomy has its roots in Enlightenment political theory and is particularly evident in the work of John Locke (1980). The consent of citizens to their government formed the basis for legitimating governmental action. By consenting, citizens became the ultimate authors of governmental action. The sovereignty of the people simply means that they have consented to and so authorize the laws through a contractual agreement. This contractual view assumes that individuals as citizens are autonomous, rational decision makers capable of consenting to be governed. As conceived in Enlightenment political theory, a theory that forms the roots of modern liberal thought, the concept of autonomy involves independence of action, speech, and thought. The ideals implicit in this concept include independence and self-determination, the ability to make rational and free decisions, and the ability to identify accurately one's own desires and preferences as well as to assess what constitutes one's own best interest. In this view, an autonomous person is by definition capable of free action and rational choice. Such abilities provide the foundation for building the social world from the myriad and motley individual beliefs, desires, preferences, and values of persons. Little consideration is given to the idea that beliefs, desires, preferences, and values might also be socially derived or influenced. Except for considering the ways that beliefs or actions can be imposed on unwilling individuals by the use of force, this line of thought views individuals in isolation from one another. Decision making is regarded as a rational process that involves the weighing of alternatives against a personal hierarchy of preferences, and communication between individuals is thought to involve primarily, if not exclusively, an exchange of information. These assumptions about the nature of persons constitute a rather large pill to swallow. They represent a view of autonomy that flies in the face of commonsense experience, which is probably why most accounts wash down this pill with copious drafts of theory.

One way to appreciate the difficulties that these assumptions create for long-term care is to point out that one central question is involved in the debate over this political theory, namely, what constitutes consent to be governed? Does consent of individuals to a political order have to be explicit or can it be tacit? A parallel debate has occurred in medical ethics regarding whether legitimate medical intervention requires explicit consent recorded by the patient's signing consent forms or whether the patient's simply having placed herself in the care of the physician constitutes a tacit consent to whatever the doctor deems necessary provided it accords with standards of care (O'Neill 1984: 174). Those who have argued that informed consent is appropriate in medical practice sometimes explicitly reject the contractual model that underlies the standard justification of informed consent. William F. May's distinction between contractual and covenant ethics in medicine is a classic statement of this debate (1975). The action-oriented ethic influenced by Enlightenment political theory assumes an idealized view of individuals as autonomous. The person is an autonomous, rational individual who functions as a discrete and isolated center of self-interested decision making. Such an individual is assumed to possess what Mill (1978: 9) called *the maturity of their faculties*. Other well-known idealizations of human rationality, such as *rational economic man*, consenting adult, cosmopolitan citizen, or *rational chooser*, similarly exhibit the tendency to regard the phenomenon of human autonomy as a matter of *ideal* rational decision making.

A different but equally influential source for abstract approaches to autonomy is Kant's account of moral agency. According to the standard, but vastly oversimplified, interpretation of Kant, the moral agent is a primarily formal and abstract construct. The moral agent autonomously wills a particular action without influence of desire and inclination, guided by a maxim or rule in which the particular contingent conditions of decision making are universalized. Such a view is undoubtedly prominent in some of Kant's ethical works, but the extent and significance of this formalism are much overstated. Nevertheless, the standard view takes Kant's conception of moral agency to be formal and abstract. On both the Kantian as well as the Lockean treatments of moral agency, an ideal moral agent is envisaged who is defined to have full rationality and freedom. The problem with both approaches is that wherever cognitive or decision-making capacities are reduced, paternalism apparently must be permissible. Both opposition to and support for paternalism in medicine rely on and reflect a remarkably abstract and relatively inaccurate view of both autonomy and the ethical processes involved in respecting autonomy.

Curiously, this entire line of thought encourages combining concern for human autonomy with (weak) paternalistic interventions. The strength of the objection to paternalism relies on the presence of distinctive cognitive and volitional capacities; their absence in frail and impaired elders thus supports a rather broad interventionist attitude that overlooks any less than ideal autonomy that might be present. Weak paternalism thus hardly provides a middle-ground solution for long-term care (Collopy 1986: 18). Having reasoned that some procedure would be consented to by an *ideally* autonomous elder, we may feel its imposition on an actual elder, who exhibits a compromised autonomy, is warranted. By shifting the focus from what has (actually) been consented to or accepted by the elder to what an elder would (ideally) consent to, actual autonomy is overridden (O'Neill 1984: 175).

Discussions of paternalism in medicine often utilize what has been termed paradigmatic four-alarm cases that shift attention from concrete, complex decision making to straightforward *in principle* moral conflicts whose resolution seems to be pre-decided by the very facts of the case. For example, bioethics discussions often feature extreme cases of patient autonomy, like the competent Jehovah's Witnesses being transfused against their expressed refusal, the lucid and rational severe burn victim being denied release from the hospital, or adult, competent patients having their dying prolonged by high-technology interventions rather than being allowed to die with dignity (McCullough and Wear 1985: 296–7). These cases are usually taken to be paradigms of medical paternalism, because they involve an interference with basic expressions of the patient's freedom. On closer inspection, however, they often involve autonomy exercised to protect or assert basic *moral concerns* of the individuals involved – the Jehovah's Witnesses' religious beliefs about blood or, in the other cases, fundamental beliefs and values about the use of life-sustaining technology at the end of life. These cases are actually about respect for the individual's basic moral concerns or values and not simply about *any* choices or decisions that an individual happens to make. Freedom from interference is understandably claimed when the issue concerns basic or fundamental beliefs or values, but this condition is not typically retained as the point is generalized to apply to other kinds of everyday cases in which basic moral concerns are not at stake in the same way (McCullough and Wear 1985: 297).

If basic beliefs and values are important elements in respecting the autonomy of even seriously incapacitated individuals, then these beliefs and values need to be identified. How they are identified is an important problem if we are concerned with the concrete conditions of autonomy in long-term care. The common tendency, however, is to avoid this question. By focusing on the incapacity or frailty of the elder, abstract action-oriented theories sanction paternalism or, worse, neglect. This tendency explains why treatment of autonomy in long-term care often focuses on discrete decision-making conflicts involving decisions to institutionalize patients or to institute, withhold, or withdraw high-technology, usually life-sustaining treatment. These situations readily lend themselves to idealization and often involve patients' actual (or imputed) basic moral beliefs or values. Such four-alarm cases distract bioethics from the broad range of everyday problems involving autonomy that does not fit this pattern.

Coupled with the political/legal lineage of the standard view of autonomy, freedom from interference has become a nearly absolute principle in bioethics; it becomes a Nozickian side-constraint (Engelhardt 1982) that focuses attention to situations of moral crises or conflict. Such a view assumes that the caregiver is a *moral* stranger to the patient and that the two share no common moral ground. If these assumptions are wrong or simply do not apply in particular cases, then freedom from interference will turn out to be a superficial and problematic interpretation of respect for autonomy.

The concrete view of persons

Autonomy involves more than explicit decision making in cases involving fundamental conflicts over moral beliefs or values. Consistent with the abstract approach discussed above, choice has been the focus of most ethical analysis, especially in the exercise of basic moral beliefs. Actual everyday consent is far more complex and involves more of values and beliefs than is generally appreciated. The practical difficulty with standard treatments of informed consent is engendered by the uncritical commitment to an abstract view of persons and the consent process. Fortunately, the legalistic understanding of consent is not the only option. One could regard, for example, informed consent as a process rather than an event (Lidz, Appelbaum, and Meisel 1988), which aims at reaching a shared understanding through communication. The event model of obtaining consent treats medical decision making as a discrete act that takes place in a circumscribed period of time, usually just before administration of treatment. The model emphasizes providing information to patients at that time. The law of informed consent has typically focused on the validity and adequacy of the disclosure and shied away from considering whether patients actually understand what they have been told and whether they accept the treatment or not. This model is consistent with the liberal theory of autonomy in which individuals are conceived as independent, rational decision makers. Because competence of patients is assumed, the professional obligation is reduced to providing accurate and complete information to allow for the informed decisions that are needed to justify the intrusion that treatment of the patient's illness involves.

An alternative model views consent as a process that is integrated into the physician–patient relationship. Consent becomes a facet of all stages of communication with patients. Loren Pankratz and Lial Kofoed (1988) helpfully describe some of the problems and pitfalls in dealing with *geezers* and discuss ways of dealing with these individuals that promote an appreciation for their rich life histories and idiosyncratic charm. They suggest that if eccentric older men are approached with interest, understanding, and respect, then half the battle is won. The conflict that these individuals tend to create can be avoided. Such an approach implies a view of personal autonomy that acknowledges the concrete experiential and social situation of persons.

Actual consent is consent to a proposed action or project *under a particular description*. To consent to an action does not mean that we consent to its logical implications or to its probable or actual results (O'Neill 1984: 174–5). In philosophical terms, consenting is, like other propositional attitudes, opaque. In consent, we are not automatically able to see through to the implications of that to which we give consent. An abstractly conceived decision maker might be able to see all the implications of a choice; but no finite agent can. To require this ability for patients generally and for those needing long-term care in particular is to force the reality to fit the theory. O'Neill has argued that consent in medical contexts is not very different from consent in other areas of life, so informed consent for medical treatment does not pose any special difficulty, but actually provides exemplary cases that highlight the typical limits associated with human autonomy in actual decision making (1984: 175). The limitations associated with actual autonomy are precisely the norm, though these limitations are insufficiently reflected in accounts of respect for autonomy guided by theories that feature an ideal view of autonomy. Rather than treating them as aberrations from ideal autonomy, concrete expressions of human autonomy need to be the focus of analysis in their own right.

O'Neill's discussion of actual autonomy focused on consent and decision making. For example, she insisted that whatever can be made comprehensible to and refusable by patients can be treated as subject to their consent or refusal. This understanding of autonomy requires physicians and other health care professionals to take time to establish effective communication with individuals in socially alienating environments. She said, 'Without such care in imparting information and proposing treatment the "consent" patients give to their treatment will lack autonomous character which would show that they have not been treated paternally but rather as persons' (O'Neill 1984: 175). In long-term care, however, treatment is not an easily delineated activity; it permeates all daily activities. Therapy potentially affects the totality of the mundane existence of individuals in long-term care. For this reason, talk about discrete treatments to which patients can be asked to consent, if only appropriate information were given, itself constitutes an idealization that inaccurately reflects the realities of long-term care.

O'Neill, however, did indicate that when we recognize the limited autonomy of actual patients, consent to all aspects and descriptions of proposed treatment is neither possible nor required. Instead, we should focus on the more fundamental actions and practices: 'Respect for autonomy requires that consent be possible to *fundamental* aspects of actions and proposals, but allows that consent to trivial and ancillary aspects of action and proposals may be absent or impossible' (O'Neill 1984: 176). Unfortunately, she did not tell us how to identify what constitutes fundamental as opposed to peripheral policies, practices, or actions. The problem is that if one makes such determination without reference to the actual autonomy of the elders involved, then paternalism will be unavoidable. If consent is focused on specific interventions, then talk of actual or concrete autonomy beyond the mere exercise of choice becomes vacuous. It is not obvious why explicit consent is *always* relevant for determining what values or courses of action ethically ought to be pursued.

These concerns have led some to commend communitarianism insofar as it provides a set of norms that can define what one ought to do, what one ought to consent to, independent of individual choice or action. We have discussed that position sufficiently in Chapter 2 to establish that it is not a viable alternative for long-term care, though features of communitarian thought will be preserved in any robust account of actual autonomy. Some components of the communitarian view, such as its insistence that human persons are fundamentally social in nature, are worth retaining. To do so, however, an account of autonomy that places human agency in its proper social nexus is needed.

Although O'Neill's discussion of actual autonomy is limited to treatment of informed consent, her discussion does point toward a more adequate account. She correctly argues that philosophical defenses of autonomy that are predicated on accounts of human rationality and decision making typically fail to come to terms with the actual range of autonomy involved in medical settings. As Bart Collopy noted, 'such defenses of autonomy lack the empirical savvy to convince and affect medical practitioners' (1986: 27). Collopy also correctly observed that O'Neill's proposal for a contextually sensitive ethic that would protect the patient as agent even while acknowledging the frequently imperfect nature of that agency would be highly relevant for frail elders:

> An action-oriented defense of autonomy would not only have to construct a defense of autonomy in the midst of impairment as O'Neill suggests; it would also have to challenge the priority given to benefit over freedom, the defining of 'benefit' primarily in medical terms, the defining of 'maximal autonomy' by caregivers rather than patients, the imbalances of power within the physician–patient relationship, and the shrinkage of patient agency in the face of high-technology, high-expertise medicine. As this agenda indicates, arguing for autonomy will mean arguing against a powerful mainstream in medicine. (Collopy 1986: 27)

This assessment is essentially correct as a reading of both O'Neill's approach and the general problems associated with providing a concrete action-centered theory of autonomy. Although Collopy stressed the difficulties facing this line of argument, he failed to note the advantages that such an account promises for an ethic of long-term care, such as forcing attention from dramatic, conflictual cases to more typical, day-to-day encounters in which the question of moral responsibility and style of practice of health professionals become central concerns. These would not be insignificant gains.

One main difficulty that any attempt to focus on actual autonomy must face is the rather messy incompleteness and uncertainty that actual autonomy inevitably involves when compared with ideal autonomy. One is forced to say something definite about when specific expressions of autonomy are genuine and when they are spurious or misleading. One cannot simply rely on hypothetical examples of ideally autonomous action or choice (i.e., action or choice taken as ideally rational and free), but rather one needs to identify specific concrete features that contribute to or mark an action or choice as being properly seen as autonomous. The problem is that autonomy is developmentally and socially conditioned, so determinate expressions of autonomy will involve unique and contextually situated assessments, thus precluding adequate formulation in abstract terms. For these reasons, a phenomenological approach that eschews theory is required. The goal of such an account is to provide a general framework for understanding autonomy in the actual contexts and circumstances of long-term care. A framework is not a theory. It may provide the scaffolding for a theory of long-term care, but a phenomenology of actual autonomy primarily aims at providing a description of the essential features that mark out autonomy in the everyday world. Taking actual autonomy seriously entails that ethical analysis be contextual and irremediably particular. To do so, we have to appreciate the prerequisites of autonomy in its everyday, interstitial expressions rather than in the conflictual nodes that are the focus of the majority of ethical analysis (Agich 1995a).

Autonomy: a developmental perspective

A theory of autonomy predicated on a concrete understanding of the person must incorporate the developmental aspects of human personhood (Haworth 1986). The idea of human development implies an end state toward which change in personal human life is directed. Jaber F. Gubrium and David R. Buckholdt point out that physical growth provides a ready model for the development of psychosexual, cognitive, affective, and moral aspects of the person. Development proceeds from relative simplicity to greater complexity of structure and differentiation of function (1977: 126). Despite the many differences among theories and approaches, contemporary ideas of human development and maturation share remarkably similar views of what it means to be immature and mature. Studies of childhood development and socialization begin with what everybody already knows, namely, that there is change in human behavior that can be differentially evaluated, depending on whether or not it appears to be moving in the proper direction toward greater maturity, rationality, and responsibility.

Scientists who study human growth and development assume that development is something real and factual, an objective theme open to scientific analysis. Contrasting terms such as adult/child, mature/immature, competent/incompetent, development/retardation as well as the idea of an order of stages in the cycle of life are likewise assumed. The resulting theories of development are thus anchored in commonsense views of human growth and change. The widespread acceptance by scientists and lay persons of the importance of certain ideas, such as life change or maturity, has glossed over the actual dynamic social processes by which change or lack of change is defined, evaluated, and shared by people in the everyday world (Gubrium and Buckholdt 1977: 129–30).

The end state or standard of human growth and development is frequently referred to by the term *maturity*. Human development is not a pyramid built from its base in infancy. Instead, development hangs from the vertex of maturity, a point toward which progress is traced. Changes in the definition or understanding of maturity thus do not simply change the description of the highest stage; they recast the entire process of development (Gilligan 1982: 18–19). Maturity and other key concepts deriving from the everyday, commonsense world are essentially historical and social in nature. Christie W. Kiefer argued that all developmental ideals are culture dependent: 'Perhaps the best example of this is the dependency of Piagetian cognitive development, and the moral conclusions drawn from it by Kohlberg, on an aesthetics that places the generality and consistency of belief at a higher level than ad hoc judgment' (Kiefer 1988: 5).

Lawrence Kohlberg's theory characterized mature moral reasoning as based on a deontological appeal to universal principles or rules that are oriented toward respecting the rights of other persons. Carol Gilligan criticized Kohlberg's results as one-sided, because his research was based exclusively on studies of males. Her own work with female subjects yielded a strikingly different model of moral maturity and the concept of autonomy. For Kohlberg, autonomy and moral maturity express dominant cultural beliefs about individual freedom and autonomy as independence, whereas Gilligan's research showed that other beliefs and values like responsibility and judgment play central roles in concrete moral choice. The debate has led to interest in distinguishing a masculine and a feminist ethic (Friedman 1989; Grimshaw 1988; Held 1987; Kittay 1999; Lerner 1986: 26; Mackenzie and Stoljar 2000; Rest et al. 1974; Saxton 1981), even though the distinction between concepts of rights and responsibilities or between an ethic of obligation and an ethic of caring seems to capture a good deal of what is at stake philosophically (Benhabib 1987; Friedman 1987; Gilligan 1987; Grimshaw 1988; Kittay and Meyers 1987; Mackenzie and Stoljar 2000; Meyers 1987; Sher 1987). This debate has brought new attention to common activities such as childrearing and parenting that are injecting valuable ideas into contemporary ethical discussion (O'Neill and Ruddick 1979). The questions about the meaning of human development and why we take it seriously are important components of the larger practical question about who we are (Kiefer 1988: 93).

The term development in our culture refers to something that is orderly, predictable, and unavoidable under usual or normal circumstances. Although development involves unspecified changes, the changes are not circular or oscillating but linear; they involve an increase rather than a decrease in those qualities that we take to be important or ideal for the person in question. In other words, decay is not a form of development. Without an idea of an ideal end state, however, processes are simply regarded as change, not development. Because we typically assume that time is linear and not cyclical, and that nature is ordered, rather than idiosyncratic or person-like, we also assume a corresponding end state that manifests order and fixity. Other cultures, however, do not share these assumptions.

In the nonliterate societies, for example, consciousness is not regarded as something amenable to development; it simply is. The idea that consciousness develops would strike people in such cultures as utterly anomalous and astounding. Individuals who fail to achieve a mature state of consciousness are thought to have been interfered with deliberately from the outside by some other consciousness or agency in a way that distorted the natural tendencies of the affected individuals (Keifer 1988: 94–5). For these reasons, Keifer (1988) argued that it is important to understand the ideal(s) associated with maturity, if maturation as a form of development is to be understood. Determining the end of human development thus is essential for defining the entire trajectory of human life and existence.

Gubrium and Buckholdt (1977: 1–31) distinguish seven different kinds of conventional – conventional in the sense that they are based on popular beliefs about the reality of life change – approaches to the question of maturity. These approaches share an uncritical belief that human growth and development are not so much a concept as an objective reality in the world of everyday life. With this acceptance comes the notion that the ideal of development, however it is articulated, is anchored in reality and so is open to scientific investigation. One might adopt a different approach, what Gubrium and Buckholdt term a social phenomenological approach. This approach sees the employment of terms such as competence, maturity, and mastery as elements in and products of a variety of social acts of interpretation that they call *negotiation*. The meaning of these terms results in a social process of negotiation around concrete problems of interpreting the behavior and development of individuals. Talk of a developmental perspective points to the fact that human persons engage in various interpretive processes or negotiations in which developmental terms acquire their meaning and reality and that these processes are themselves described and defined in various theories that are broadly called developmental. Understanding human development as a process of the social construction of meaning is highly relevant to our focus on actual autonomy. Cultural values and social interpretations shape the reality of long-term care and delineate the conditions under which we are able to see autonomy at work.

Autonomy, as it concretely emerges in the practical world of everyday life as opposed to the ideal world of theory, necessarily involves processes of interpretation and negotiation. So to adopt a developmental perspective on autonomy is to ask how is autonomy established in the world of everyday life through concrete interpretive processes. If autonomy is not an ideal state defined in ethical theory, it must represent a rather broad set of attributes or capabilities that all or most members of society exhibit. Included in this way of framing the concept of autonomy, of course, will be normative elements that involve both individual perceptions and social perceptions of each mature individual. A dominant set of norms that are especially relevant to autonomy involve independence and self-sufficiency. Underlying these norms is an assumption that human growth and development achieve some determinate end state that yields a finished product, namely, an independent, competent, rational, and free decision maker. These norms are taken for granted to such an extent that they resist analysis in many everyday contexts. Consider, for instance, the kinds of circumstances in which maturity is commonly an issue.

Questions of competence arise in circumstances characterized by dispute, disagreement, or conflict. In the practice of medicine, decision-making capacity is usually not an issue when patients consent or passively accept a proposed intervention, but when they refuse to follow the doctor's recommendations. Similarly, the question of competence is raised in other social situations such as when one party in a divorce challenges the spouse's ability and right to care for the children. In many, if not most, social contexts, competence becomes an issue when important matters are at stake. Questions of competence in the context of long-term care are judged in terms of an elder's rationality, reality orientation, or decisional abilities; they usually arise when there is disagreement over the proper care or welfare of the elder. An important subject for investigation thus concerns the concrete circumstances, and the typical ways that autonomy is attributed to elders in need of long-term care reflect unfounded attitudes or biases.

The literature on the concept of human development provides strong evidence that attitudes toward elders are socially shaped. This is not surprising, since sociality is an essential feature of human existence. Without social life and intact processes of socialization, the emergence of an intact individual as a biopsychosocial unity capable of thought and action would be impossible. Indeed, social life makes autonomy, no matter how we define it, possible, because without the social world there would be no space for agency. Human action acquires its meaning in and through the social world. Emphasizing social life, however, does not make autonomy an ethically derivative or secondary concern as familiar criticisms of communitarian approaches assume. As pointed out in Chapter 2, one can acknowledge the social nature of human existence and autonomy without embracing specific metaphysical commitments about the self or communitarian commitments to tradition and community as a foundation for authority. Rather, attention to the social nature of action points us away from an abstract consideration of autonomy and toward concrete estimation of actual developmental processes.

Attention to the social character of human development forces the realization that dependence is an essential feature of human existence and that autonomy must be reinterpreted to accommodate social arrangements such as family, friendship, and community associations that make possible autonomous human existence in the first place. Dependence is therefore problematic not in itself, but in juxtaposition to an abstract ideal of autonomy as negative freedom. Viewed positively, however, autonomy involves a dialectic of independence and dependence that takes place with a social space characterized by interdependence. Dependence consequently ceases to be a universal problem to be erased or resolved, but becomes particularized in situations and circumstances, some of which may enhance or efface autonomy.

The liberal concept of autonomy focuses on independence and self-control and prescribes noninterference as a primary value. Independence and self-control each point to different features of autonomy. These are common delineations of autonomy. There is, however, a more fundamental dimension of personal autonomy. This dimension underlies the various social attributions of competence as a fully autonomous agent. Both independence and self-control qualify behavior, but simply being able to act is itself an achievement that is highly relevant to considerations of autonomy. As Lawrence Haworth pointed out:

No one begins life as an agent. When for the first time the corners of an infant's mouth turn up, the infant isn't smiling. The first time the rattle falls from his hand he isn't dropping the rattle. Agency is an acquired ability. By exercising the ability, the infant builds a repertoire of performances appropriate for various needs and occasions. He learns how to get his mouth to the nipple, how to get attention, how to stand and walk. 'Competence' presupposes the ability to act and refers to the adequacy of the repertoire.
    The root phenomenon is the trying (undertaking, endeavoring) . . . 'Trying,' in turn, is the root of 'intending.' (1986: 13)

Passing from barely trying to full-fledged intending involves bringing into focus what one is trying to accomplish. Haworth argued that by barely trying the infant establishes himself as a minimal agent. The development of competence beyond this level consists in becoming able to produce intended effects. In this way, he traces the beginnings of autonomy back to the individual's first signs of competence as an agent. The competence at issue is admittedly minimal, indeed nascent, but nonetheless crucial to an adequate understanding of autonomy in the context of long-term care.
    Haworth argues that humans possess a basic competence motive, a motive that involves the effort to be an agent, to gain control over one's environment, beyond this, to expand control by developing both a specific repertoire of skills and a generalized coping ability (1986: 55; White 1959, 1960). He points out that maintaining this minimum sense of competence is the infant's first project; the ability to do so often against odds strongly suggests that the disposition to do so is part of the equipment that the individual brings on entering the world. As a wide range of work in developmental psychology has shown, this disposition is a general or universal human potentiality (Haworth 1986: 55).
    The competence motive and the phenomenon of trying are important not as abstract conditions, but because of the inescapably particular and determinate way that they are manifested in individual lives. Autonomy is not a logically necessary outcome of human development from infancy onward, but rather an empirical and altogether perilous process of achievement that occurs in dynamic interaction with others. To be autonomous is to be a particular agent individualizing oneself in particular circumstances through effortful striving

in the shared social world. The striving, however, does not have an ideal of autonomy as some pre-given and logically assured end state; rather, such striving is itself autonomy in an inchoate or nascent form. The striving may take many forms, because individuals are unique. As individuals mature, their competencies are achieved in their unique biographical circumstances. As a result, the expression of autonomy is unique in each individual's life. Saying this does not mean that human autonomy does not exhibit patterns, but that the patterns are achieved in each individual's biography.

For these reasons, autonomy should not be regarded as an end state of being or stage of development that can be achieved once and for all, but as a precarious achievement that is actively maintained as agents engaged with the world. To be autonomous is to be bound not only to others and history, but to the forces of contingency and luck (Nussbaum 1986). Autonomy is thus not a metaphysical given or an end state, but the complex process of interpretation or negotiation that is the hallmark of how individuals actually live their lives. Paradoxically, autonomy is based on an achieved or sedimented sense of self. The self is never abstract, but is a particular and determinate entity engaging in the world. To think of autonomy as a state or an autonomous subject as an accomplished entity is thus to adopt a conventional perspective that obscures more than it reveals. To speak *simply* of autonomy is inevitably to speak elliptically, if not misleadingly.

The autonomy of a so-called developed or mature self consists not simply in the achievement of an end state, but in the use of a particular repertoire of skills and abilities, desires and preferences that are themselves the products of past efforts and enactments in the world. All of these abilities or capacities are subject to interpretation by others in the complex dynamic that comprises the world of everyday life. Autonomy fundamentally involves striving and experiencing the world in a precarious dialectic of habit and choice.

Narrative approaches

Consideration of autonomy in long-term care requires that we think about actual agents in the world. How we think about actual autonomy is not a tangential concern. The language of general abilities or commitments employed in developmental psychology is inevitably abstract, so we should not rely on this terminology. A more appropriate way to view the development and meaning of actual autonomy involves narrative and story. Because personal identity always involves the biography of a unique person, it is presupposed by the concept of personal autonomy (Dworkin 1993: 205; Quante 2000). Thus, biographical narrative becomes an indispensable mode of access into the phenomenon of personal autonomy. This philosophical insight has a parallel in the growing interest in biography, life review, life story, and reminiscence in gerontological circles (Baum 1980–81; Berman 1994; Butler 1963, 1980–81; Johnson 1976;

Kaminsky 1984; Merriam 1980; Moody 1984a; Rich 1996; Woodward 1986). As elders relate their life stories, they actively rearrange and reconstitute memories as a way of establishing location and direction in the (sometimes alien) present world of experience. Such an activity is an important manifestation of the actual autonomy of the elder to give meaning to her life and to make her present experiences meaningful.

Biographical construction, and indeed reconstruction since the process of telling and retelling stories about oneself involves creative adaptation to new circumstances, occurs on many different occasions. This truth seems to have escaped many in that people seem to regard the past as something that objectively happened to the individual up to the present. On this typical understanding, biography is assumed primarily, if not exclusively, to be a matter for discovery. It would seem that an elder's story is a story that anyone with access to the relevant facts could tell. Such an interpretation is very far from the truth. In telling the story of one's life or writing someone's biography, one needs to do more than search out what really happened to the individual in the past. On this view, the elder is not seen in a unique or privileged position with respect to the construction of the life story.

There are at least two elements involved in knowing somebody's past: the past and the knower. Emphasis is conventionally placed on the past (Gubrium and Buckholdt 1977: 158–91). The knower is tacitly assumed to be a passive net that gathers the facts of the past or, at worse, as someone who distorts what really happened. Once it is taken for granted that an individual has a real past that occurred and is knowable, it becomes mostly a technical affair to gain insight into someone's past, personal history, or life story. On this conventional or typical view, then, biography is an objective depiction of an elder's life story. The other element of the equation, namely, that biography is the product of work done by the biographer, is less commonly appreciated. Biographies are constructed and they serve complex social purposes.

Usually, people take it for granted that biography is always singular and individual. The fact that individuals can and do tell different stories about themselves under different circumstances and at different phases of life (Goffman 1963) is not readily appreciated. Given the assumption that biography is single, incompatible stories are explained away by reconstructing a new life story in terms of new facts, once the new facts are accepted as real. So, for example, a politician's career can be reinterpreted once his homosexuality is revealed. Thenceforward, the entire past is given a new, but now taken as the *true*, rendition. As Gubrium and Buckholdt pointed out:

Biographical work is a search for integrating accounts that lead to overall intelligibility. This process of integration requires a good deal of glossing, because the biography being considered is always the biography at hand. In someplace, at sometime, an individual's past is being considered. This limitation in space and time is meaningful to biographers in that the tacit background of specific situations defines 'relevant' biography. (1977: 161)

This process is nowhere more evident in long-term care than in the way that the details of elders' lives are glossed over and explained in terms of their cognitive impairments or the label of Alzheimer's. Leaving aside whether these terms have any particular diagnostic validity in particular cases, the fact that an individual's life can be so readily reconstituted and reduced through the foreshortening perspective that such labels create raises obvious questions about the effect of biography on autonomy in long-term care.

In contrast to the conventional assumptions about biography, life stories can be regarded as matters that are not objective or open for discovery at all, but rather are constructed through elaborate interpretive processes. On this view, the past is not simply out there, but exists only as the storyteller constitutes it in the present. The past is what the biographer produces by reflecting on the given facts in such a way that they are made intelligible for present purposes. Constructing a biography or telling one's life story is thus a constructive, interpretive process. It involves the conferral of meaning about oneself and the whole of one's life course. Thus, when individuals tell stories about themselves, each story represents an effort to make sense of the present in light of a constructed or invented past. One's past, in this view, is not an independent reality or truth in itself, but is a phenomenon constituted in the present to make sense of things for some storyteller or biographer.

Constructing a biography is, therefore, an important social action that occurs in long-term care as in other areas of social life. The importance of formal records in institutional long-term care, for example, creates a medically oriented biography of the institutionalized elder's life course not only in the nursing home, but previously. Charting the care that elders receive is thus essentially an interpretive project that places the elder in an interpretive framework that largely excludes the elder's own sense of herself. Efforts to correct this dominance of the medical biography have turned toward life story and reminiscence as significant ways to integrate the elder as a person into this important social process. These efforts sometimes miss the mark if they overlook the informal record of the elders' lives that is embodied in their personal possessions, their photographs, and even their clothes. Many of these objects are links to the person's life story and can be used in helping elders to maintain links with their past as they struggle with infirmities in the present.

One can, of course, celebrate a life story or a biography from a distance, omitting any real linkage with the person. A story, even a life story, is not really the person, so it may prove much easier and more comfortable to deal with the actual person. One danger associated with the fascination with narrative and story in gerontology is that it can displace the existential engagement with the person in long-term care. That danger, however, is counterbalanced by the positive effects of attending to the life story that are corollary to the interest in narrative. Stories involve and are about persons who deserve respect in the present. It is, of course, wrong to revel in some particular elder's life story as if it were a novel open to the hermeneutic gaze without a keen awareness of the person's needs, motives, and purposes, latent though they may be, in telling the story. For these reasons, interest in life stories does not itself assure that the autonomy of elders will be respected. If attending to the stories of elders achieves respect for elders by increasing the awareness of caregivers to the unique identity of elders, by teaching the young generally about the rich complexity of old age, or by making specific individuals sensitive to the actual needs of particular elders, then the gerontological emphasis on narrative and life story is laudable.

Stories, however, are artifices once removed from the events they recount that gerontologists, like all academics, are prone to celebrate in place of the reality that they not only convey, but also necessarily displace. The ethical significance of actual autonomy in long-term care is not to celebrate being old and infirm from afar, but rather to close the gaps with elders in long-term care. The significant point about stories is that what people tell about their lives comprises one of the most important modes of access to what is important to them. Stories drawn from one's life can indicate the things that people value most; they tell us who the person is and with what they most identify. For stories to function in this way, however, caregivers must listen and be open to story telling as an important caregiving function. Making an elder's life meaningfully available to caregivers – or, better still, making caregivers capable of hearing an elder's stories – is an important way to assure that a central practical concern of actual autonomy will be achieved.

Stories, however, invite, if not require, interpretation, and the interpretive process needs to be open to the elder's own revisions. The hermeneutic of an elder's life story, or any particular story told by an elder for that matter, does not belong to specialists but to those who know the elder best, ultimately, the elder herself. Stories are open only to those who are close enough to the elder to listen and hear. This is one practical reason justifying the use of family surrogates for decision making when the elder loses decisional ability, because they probably know the elder best. Constructing a biography points out how our present actions, choices, and experiences, no matter how free and rational they appear, never float in a vacuum as philosophers like Sartre (1966) picture autonomy, but reflect the achieved competencies and abilities that define the particular individual's self-identify, an identity that is itself essential in process and not fixed.

Dependence in human development

The interesting and important problem posed by dependence is not in abstract cases in which it appears to constrain the free exercise of will abstractly regarded, but in contexts of actual choice and experience. The view that will or freedom in pursuing one's desires or preferences is fundamental is an understandable outcome of a model of autonomy that abstracts from concrete life. Will, desire, and preference are not the fundamental phenomenological features of autonomy. Theoretical treatments of desire do not significantly help us to apprehend, much less to fathom, the nuanced phenomena of an individual's actual autonomy.

Humans develop through relationships with significant others such as parents. They do not simply exist in some pristine theoretical space as competent, rational, and independent decision makers. The relationships necessary for human development are made possible not primarily by will, since it is through them that will itself emerges, but by affectivity that binds parent and child and individuals with each other in the everyday world. Such feeling for fellow humans is not just an ideal of moral character, but a feature necessary to being a person in the world. Individuals instinctively reach out to others and the world, because the intentional nature of consciousness involves an openness to the world. Reciprocal affective connections constitute one of the conditions essential for human individuality. Such connections are essential to developing what psychoanalysts call object relations, namely, relations with the world and reality.

Affections determine who we are. This view has support in the accepted understanding of human growth and development. Formation of the rational will from primitive desires or preferences occurs only in relationship with others, relations that are made possible through bonds of affection (Bowlby 1969, 1973, 1980). Affectivity and not will is primary to the process of developing autonomy. It is at least as important as desire, because it provides the nurturing nexus for the fulfillment and objectification of desire. Affectivity is the means by which a rational will developmentally emerges. Consideration of human development thus necessarily brings forward the social and historical nature of human life. Actual autonomy can be assessed only in a framework that takes these factors seriously.

One main problem with mainstream treatments of the faculty of will as a fundamental expression of autonomy is the way that attention to choice and decision making has effaced the wider context of conation. Desire, too, is treated as a relatively determinant phenomenon involving discrete objects amenable to cognitive expression. What these approaches omit, however, is of central concern for assessing the significance of autonomy in long-term care, especially for cognitively impaired or confused elders. Many treatments of autonomy ask the question 'What does autonomy mean?', rather than the question 'What is it like to be autonomous?' or 'In what does autonomy actually consist?'. These philosophical treatments have focused primarily on the concept or definition of autonomy. In treating autonomy and long-term care, however, the question 'What is involved in respecting people's autonomy?' should be primary. Focusing on this question makes autonomy conceived as negative freedom almost irrelevant and instead brings to the forefront the related questions 'What does it mean to be an agent in the world?' or 'What does it mean to feel confused, incapacitated, or vulnerable?' or 'What features of everyday experience structure the expression or manifestation of autonomy in action?'.

Human life and, hence, human development are essentially phenomena that involve interdependence. Individuals develop as human persons not simply because biological needs are fulfilled, but because psychosocial needs are also met. Consider the following thought experiment. By means of in-vitro fertilization, a human embryo is created and allowed to develop extracorporeally. Also, imagine the availability of an artificial womb capable of sustaining the developing embryo through the fetal development to the point of prenatal maturity. At term the infant is delivered into the world, that is, the infant's biological dependence on the artificial intrauterine environment is severed and the infant is able to exist as a separate biological entity in the world. At this point, imagine also that every biological need is met through a series of robotic devices that feed and wash the infant. No strictly biological need is left unmet. Would such an infant develop into a normal human person? Assume that the infant reaches childhood, adolescence, and adulthood. Would such a human being be an individual, be a person, an autonomous agent in the world? Would it even be correct to say that such an entity had a world in the sense of a distinctively human world?

Research suggests that an intact human person would not emerge under such circumstances (Bowlby 1969, 1973; Harlow and Harlow 1962; Spitz 1965). Why not? Simply put, because human development is not only biological, but psychosocial as well. What is missing from our example is the requisite psychosocial interaction. To be sure, one might imaginatively vary the case to allow the infant to view simulated faces in order to elicit the so-called social smile and permit robotic cuddling, but such modifications only delay the inevitable conclusion. Without significant interaction with some type of parents, actual caregivers, the infant would not develop into a human person, even if she could survive to adulthood. Empirical evidence suggests that there would be quite a high risk of early mortality (Spitz 1965). What would be missing would be the emergence of a set of traits, skills, and abilities, such as human language and all the components of autonomous agency: a relatively unified pattern and range of feelings, as well as a unique capacity for reasoning and will that comprise the self-identity of the person. Dependence on others is thus an essential feature of human development. Dependence is not simply a matter of privation or biological need, but an essential condition of what it means to be a human person as an integrated biopsychosocial entity.

Because we culturally prize independence, it is natural to view dependence of any sort as a defect. This cultural attitude distorts our understanding of human development and our interdependent existence. There are no telling senses in which human persons are not dependent on others. Even hermits are children of human parents; their cultural and social context may be forsaken, but it can never be completely eradicated, because the meaning of their thoughts and feelings is determined linguistically. Fascination throughout the centuries with the idea of a feral child can be credited not simply to a fascination with the usual or extraordinary, but also with an inchoate realization that such an entity would be a living counterexample to our universal, though usually tacit, understanding of what a human person is. Dependence in the social world is a pressing position and not a failure of actual autonomy.

Underlying the central dependence of human beings is the fact that human persons are embodied entities in the world. The human body is not only a vehicle for one's autonomous choice or will, but also an impediment. The world and other persons also resist our efforts to act in and on them. This resistance represents not simply obstacles to be overcome, but defines the fundamental sense of dependence, namely human persons *exist in the world*. Human existence involves what Martin Heidegger (1962) so aptly character-ized as *Geworfenheit*, being thrown or thrownness. Humans are thrown into the world. We find ourselves in the world and are dependent on it. Achieving maturity or old age does not lessen this fundamental existential dependence. In fact, just the opposite is true. The engaged activity that our culture views as independence and takes as characteristic of middle age obscures this more basic sense of dependence.

Dependence thus is an essential and ineliminable feature of human exis-tence. It is an obvious feature of human development, as human development is commonly conceptualized in terms of stages: infancy, childhood, adoles-cence, and adulthood. Humans, however, are never finished, but are essentially open to the future. For this reason, all human beings are dependent no matter what their stage of development. The issue of elder dependence needs to be phrased not as a problematic feature of being old and frail – since dependence as a general existential condition is not unique to class alone – but in terms of the way it uniquely is manifested in the life of particular elders. Since the general existential conditions of being in the world are not our central con-cern, we can illustrate how the essential dependence of humans in the world is exemplified in frail elders in long-term care by discussing the conditions that commonly bring elders into long-term care, namely, illness or disability.

Sickness as dependence

Illness invariably involves a dissolution of the unity of body and self. Normally in the everyday world, the self is experienced as one with one's actions. The body is simply the vehicle for achieving ends in the world and is transparent to our intentions. I am not aware of my hand as I write. I am aware of my thoughts, which are achieved by the pen in my hand in a complex process about which

I am not usually aware. In illness, dissolution occurs in the normal relationship between the self, the body, and the world.

Because of sickness, one comes to depend on others to compensate for one's physical shortcomings. This dependence is expressed in the very social world of the patient. It includes needing help to perform activities of daily living or at least to substitute for those activities that the body cannot exercise on its own. The sick person also becomes dependent in needing to rely on experts to remove or to ameliorate the first dependence. Sickness typically involves the social expectation that a professional has determined that one is legitimately in need of special care and is eligible to be exempted from normal social role activities (Parsons 1958, 1975). For the elder this exemption may not involve the world of work. The exemption instead frequently means that the elder is deemed unable or incapable, at least without undue risk to self, to carry out the normal activities of everyday life including self-care activities. Therefore, the elder is exempted from the normal world of life and experience and forced to accept assistance.

The sick elder is dependent, sometimes pervasively so, on others in a way that is atypical for most normal adults. This situation leads to experiences of loss of hope and mistrust as the sick elder has to accommodate the incapacity and the dependence on caregivers in dealing with the first dependence (Bergsma and Thomasma 1982: 177). The dependence of the frail or incapacitated elder can result in a specific infantilization as the elder finds herself needing supervision and help with basic activities of daily living. In a variety of ways, the sick elder is placed in the hands of others. Given the expectation of recovery and resumption of normal social role activities associated with being sick in our society, it is a constant source of frustration for sick elders because this usually powerful expression of hope is recognized as a pallid counterfeit. Talk of recovery or doing better can understandably be perceived as mockery or ridicule by an elder who realistically fears lack of recovery.

In a sense, the world is judged and experienced by the degree and kind of care that others are willing and able to extend. It is also structured by the degree and kind of care that the sick person is willing or able to accept. This latter point is important because we sometimes think that the diagnosis determines in an objective fashion the degree or kind of help that should be offered. As pointed out in the previous chapter, this mistake is one of the systemic problems facing long-term care. There is no objective measure of seriousness of the illness. Illness is a subjectively experienced phenomenon. Largely, then, the sick elder is also dependent on the ways that others perceive the illness. When there is a discrepancy between the perceptions, when the illness for which there is no medical cure is nonetheless viewed only in medical terms, a greater chance for despair and frustration is assured (Bergsma and Thomasma 1982: 179). The problem, however, is less an issue of dependence than a matter of the meanings that dependence imposes on the particular elder.

Insofar as care is taken over by another, one becomes disengaged and alienated from the normal and everyday activities through which one relates to oneself. There is no alternative. This state of affairs is simply unavoidable. The patient thus surrenders not simply a part of her body to the caregiver or a set of activities, but an essential part of the self. That is probably why most elders, and people in general, prefer care rendered by those with whom they share bonds of affection rather than by strangers, no matter how well trained or qualified they may be. One's sense of self might be less at risk when care is rendered by people who care. It is indeed ironic that much effort is expended in trying to eliminate affect from the professional caregiving or treatment relationships, when harnessing the positive affect could help avoid job and career routinization and directly address the elder's reticence regarding care. As Julius R. Roth pointed out:

> The way to avoid job and career routinization is to put the care taking tasks into the hands of those for whom the patient is also a special case, namely the people who love him.
>
> Let us consider the matter of caring for a sick person. There are signs to watch for, perhaps equipment to check on, medicines and other treatment to give. When such care is turned over to hired hands (as it routinely is in hospitals in our society), it is scarcely surprising that a great many errors (mostly errors of omission) are made. The patient is a victim of job routinization. He is not the special case of anyone who has his interest primarily at heart. He is dependent on people who will tend to him if they remember, if they consider it appropriate to their job, if he has not demanded 'too much' from them already, and if they do not have too much else to do. Here indeed is affective neutrality at work with scarcely inspiring results. (1973: 175)

A tension always exists between self and body, but in everyday life, the world experienced is the tenuous unity of self and body. Disruption of this unity lurks at the edge of every action and perception. The continuity of experience is always under threat. Hence, anxiety lies at the root of our everyday existence. Alfred Schutz (1967, 1970) has argued that a fundamental anxiety regarding death and finitude underlies all our actions in the social world. This anxiety explains our readiness to engage the world from the moment of our birth. Actual autonomy for finite persons thus consists in acting in the face of our fragile hold on existence and the world around us. In the world of social action, this anxiety is channeled into individual projects and actions, and so its experience is usually suppressed. It is brought forward, however, by illness, because illness accentuates the fundamental gap that exists between one's self, life, and existence in the world.

The disruption in the unity of body, self, and world occasioned by illness and disability creates an increased concern for the body. We usually take our bodies for granted. Even devotees of healthy living take their bodies for granted in the sense that they are not reflectively aware of most bodily functions and processes as they actively pursue the goal of health. The avid jogger, for example, might be motivated by the desire for cardiovascular health and fitness or the exhilaration of exercise, but is usually unaware of the effect of running on the legs, that is, until an ankle or knee injury stops this single-minded pursuit. Illness, whether caused by specific disease processes or by the normal process of aging, draws the attention of elders to their bodies. Periodic or episodic attention to the body is normal, but for most adults it is relatively confined given the episodic character of illness. Since most adults are actively engaged in the everyday world, meeting the demands of work and everyday existence, pains and discomforts are regularly discounted. The sense of illness or the feeling of something being not quite right is set aside by the active person in pursuing projects. Most adults do not have time to be sick and consequently may delay investigation or treatment of the illness or deny its occurrence. This behavior occurs when the individual is actively engaged in the social world and it seems adaptive in cases of most minor and acute illnesses.

In the case of chronic illness, however, individuals must acknowledge and accommodate themselves to the illness if they are to manage. In a sense, such individuals must actively work to modify their behaviors and expectations to accommodate the limitations imposed by chronic disease processes (Agich 1995b). Elders suffering with chronic disease naturally fixate on bodily processes. As a result, bodily signals such as fatigue or pain are given greater attention. The attention is not the neutral and disinterested gaze of an abstract consciousness, but is laden with concrete meanings and values. When the meanings are unclear, it is difficult to interpret the signals. The more suspicious the interpretations, the more uncertain and anxious the patient becomes (Bergsma and Thomasma 1982: 179).

These bodily signals, however, are not meaningful in themselves; they require interpretation. Uncertainty makes communication of information and participation in the process of identifying and interpreting the meaning of signals and symptoms by others important. There is good evidence that providing patient information, for example before surgery regarding the experiences that might be expected postoperatively, is associated with better outcomes (Lindeman and van Aernham 1971). Such communication strengthens the patients' trust not only in their own bodies, but also in the caregiver who predicted and correctly interpreted the effects (Bergsma and Thomasma 1982: 179). It is often forgotten by caregivers that the attention patients give to bodily processes is necessarily part of the interpretive effort to make sense of a fractured experience that is reduced to or focused on the body. The activity of interpretation is familiar, but the focus is strikingly different because the field of view, so to speak, is so truncated (Bergsma and Thomasma 1982: 180).

The sense of time is distorted and the past and future are squeezed into the present and modified by the overriding concern with one's symptoms. Egocentrism and dependence are compatible, though in necessary tension.

Given this tension, it is not surprising that ambivalence is a frequent result. It is often very difficult for sick elders to know whether their frustration is with the caregiver or with themselves and their situation. Frustrations also occur on the part of caregivers; it is important that caregivers distinguish their own frustrations about their own inadequacies in caring for the compromised elder from the frustrations with the elder.

A closeness or proximity develops in which the caregiver is linked with the sick elder to such a degree that it is sometimes difficult for the sick elder to distinguish herself from others. This deep practical problem is inevitable in these relationships. Failure to attend to the psychosocial aspects of the caregiving relationship makes it difficult to imagine how one could enhance the autonomy of elders in long-term care. It is far easier in a dependence relationship simply to take over the care of the elder without ever intending to return it. What prevents this usurpation of the elder's autonomy is a caring and respectful attitude toward him that is achieved by responsibly working to help him maintain his identity and autonomy despite the onslaught of impairment.

These general points about dependence in states of illness help us to understand why autonomy seems so alien a concept in long-term care. Autonomy is first a problem not because powerful caregivers or institutions limit the freedom of frail elders, as thinkers dominated by a primarily political model of autonomy would have it, but because the existential conditions that create the need for long-term care contravene autonomy as independent self-sufficiency remarkably unsuited to the purposes of concrete ethical assessment. For this purpose, another, fuller concept of autonomy is needed.

Autonomy and identification

Autonomy literally means self-rule, that is, behavior that is spontaneous and self-initiated; such behavior is regarded as action in the sense that it manifests intentionality. Human action, in turn, can be regarded as free if the individual agent can identify with the elements from which it flows; an action (or choice) is unfree or coerced if the agent cannot identify with or dissociates from the elements that generate or prompt the action (Bergmann 1977: 37). This means that identification, the ability to reflexively recognize as one's own the constituents of an action, is logically prior to freedom; autonomy is best understood on the basis of the possession of an identity or of a self having a particular determinate nature and character. Expressions of autonomy are thus enactments of who the individual is in the process of becoming. The field or stage for such playing out is the social world of everyday life.

Saying that formed identifications are the precondition for the real possibility of freedom entails a paradox. Freedom stresses the priority of the self as an individual, which is precisely what autonomy is designed to support. Given that identifications do not occur in a vacuum but are socially situated, a society can work toward establishing frameworks for the development of autonomy and the exercise of freedom, while at the same time specific institutions or social settings can exhibit patterns that thwart the expression of the self or stunt its development (Bergmann 1977: 39). The concretely, as opposed to ideally, autonomous individual is necessarily caught up in the web of contingent forces and subject to the fate or circumstances that either augment or diminish the conditions supporting autonomy (Nussbaum 1986).

Because autonomous individuals are situated in concrete social contexts, choice is always contextual. To choose x means that y is foregone. Choosing x also means that action, sometimes effortful action, is necessary to pursue the object of choice. Choice does not automatically bring into being its object. Costs are thus always associated with any choice. The explicit making of choices or decisions, however, is not the central feature of our lives; most of our lives are spent acting in habitual, taken-for-granted ways that are not experienced as explicit decision making. To be sure, it still makes sense to speak of choice, but the choice under discussion is not overt. As with choice, so with action.

Another important and basic sense of autonomy is freedom of action. Action is an engagement in the ambient world. It is embodied choice. Some actions and choices reflect habit. The traditional concept of autonomy as rational, free agency implies that free actions are the result of a deliberative process that yields a decision defensible on rational grounds. On this view, prior reflection and decision are necessary for an action to be judged as free. Is this a tenable view? As John Searle observed in another context:

We ought to allow ourselves to be struck by the implications of the fact that at any point in a man's conscious life he knows without observation the answer to the question, 'What are you now doing?' . . . Even in a case where a man is mistaken about what the results of his efforts are he still knows what he is trying to do. (1983: 90)

This intentional awareness is coextensive with action and experience; it points to the presence of an intention-in-action that is an essential feature of the prereflective self-awareness that accompanies all autonomous experience. Autonomy is thus best regarded as a phenomenon of the intentional nature of consciousness. The deficiency common to most treatments of individual autonomy is that they abstract from the phenomenological complexity of actual consciousness and treat autonomy as a one-dimensional phenomenon. On standard views, everyday actions or choices that are habitual or taken for granted are either uninteresting or regarded as unfree. Such actions and choices, however, are animated by an occurrent self-awareness that is an essential feature of consciousness. From a different point of view, one could argue that actions and choices are truly free or unfree to the extent that they are consistent with the person's self-identity. The requirement that explicit rational decision making underlie all truly free action or choice or that second-order reflection or intention must always accompany autonomous agency sets too rigorous a standard. Autonomy on such a view is an idealization that makes sense only in light of an abstract or idealized view of the self. Actual persons could not long endure the burden of analysis and deliberation that such a view implies.

For actual, as opposed to ideal, selves, autonomy always involves and relies on developed patterns. I am more autonomous because my thoughts move automatically through my fingers and into my computer, not less. The skill or habit of typing enhances and extends my autonomy rather than limits it. The relationship between what is done automatically in normal human experience and autonomy has unfortunately been effaced, as most philosophical treatments constrictively focus attention on choice and will. In a fuller sense, specific action or choices can be judged to be truly free or unfree not simply because the agent performed some particular deliberative or reflective validation, but to the extent that they are consistent with the agent's self-identity. Since individuals are always in the process of formation, 'who an individual self actually is' is always an open question for the person. Thus, the person is not a slave to the past, since present choices and actions can alter the commitments and identity of the self, but neither is a person autonomous when past associations and affiliations are alienated.

In the daily course of living, the question 'Who am I?' is typically suspended or set aside as a conscious matter for inquiry, but that does not mean the matter is ever really closed. The Socratic aphorism that an unexamined life is not worth living should not be taken as if philosophical reflection or psychological introspection was the only way in which such questions are explicitly opened. Existential crises or life transitions are clearly paradigmatic ways in which questions such as 'Who am I?' or 'In what do I believe?' come to the fore. Sickness, too, frequently forces an examination of what is so commonly termed one's values. In daily life, however, we are able to proceed quite nicely, oblivious to our own spontaneity and freedom. The daily adjustments of intentionality as our efforts are fulfilled or frustrated in the world of actual experience constitute another ever-present way that persons autonomously act in the world. Such action is not one sided, but interactive. The world exerts its inexorable demands and places limits on the scope of meaningful action. Lack of explicit reflective awareness or the cognitive ability to discuss such awareness, then, cannot be taken to imply that autonomy is not present; rather, the actual rarity of fully rational, reflective deliberation regarding courses of action and outcomes should serve to remind us of the idealized status of standard philosophical models of human autonomy. The failure of much current ethical theory to take this point seriously seems an example of what Alfred North Whitehead termed *the fallacy of misplaced concreteness*, namely, the error of mistaking the abstract for the concrete (1948: 52).

Self-identity is not something that one discovers as an uncharted island in the middle of a sea, but rather is something that is made by individuals in the very course of their living. It is less something solid than it is like a lubricant that we secrete as we slip through our lives and experiences of the world. To speak meaningfully of individuals as autonomous requires that we pay attention to the kinds of things with which individuals properly identify in their lives. Saying this is to expand on the slogan *respect for persons* in a way that reflects the concrete reality of human existence.

Frithjof Bergmann (1977: 48) nicely articulated the central elements of such a concrete concept of autonomy. He noted that it is only for those without a developed sense of identity that freedom has to mean absolute independence. Since they lack a substantive sense of self, they must oppose things in order to be free. This is not the case for individuals who do not share this extreme condition. The greater the extent to which individuals do identify with something, the less is the complete isolation requisite for their being free. To put the point paradoxically: to be dependent on something does not in any way diminish one's degree of freedom as long as one truly identifies with the thing on which one is dependent. If I am in harmony with something, if in fact it is me – and that is the point of talking about identification – then I do not need to be protected or isolated from it in order to be autonomous. The demand that autonomy be respected takes the form of an insistence on total independence only for those who lack identity or for those things with which individuals cannot identify. In other, more typical circumstances, it is unnecessary to regard autonomy in such an extreme way.

The idea that autonomy involves identification and the possession of a self-identity is even evident in Mill's classic treatment of liberty. He, too, insisted that individuals require unique and distinctive conditions for their existence:

If a person possesses any tolerable amount of common sense and experience, his own mode of laying out of his existence is the best, not because it is the best in itself, but because it is his own mode. Human beings are not like sheep; and even sheep are not undistinguishably alike. A man cannot get a coat or a pair of boots to fit him unless they are either made to his measure or he has a whole warehouseful to choose from; and is it easier to fit him with a life than with a coat, or are human beings more like one another in their whole physical and spiritual conformation than in the shape of their feet? If it were only that people have diversities of taste, that is reason enough for not attempting to shape them all after one model. But different persons also require different conditions for their spiritual development; and can no more exist healthily in the same moral than all the variety of plants can in the same physical atmosphere and climate. The same things which are helps to one person toward the cultivation of his higher nature are hindrances to another. The same mode of life is a healthy excitement to one, keeping all his faculties of action and enjoyment in their best order, while to another it is a distracting burden which suspends or crushes all internal life. (Mill 1978: 64–5)

Not only is tolerance of diversity of choice and taste a prerequisite for respecting liberty, but so is acknowledging the irreducible individuality of concrete expressions of autonomy in individuals. To be autonomous thus does not require that one be able to manifest ideally rational and reflective free choice; what is required is to have a developed identity.

Another way to make this point would be to argue, following Robert B. Young (1986), that personal autonomy is a character ideal. The character ideal of autonomy is expressed in three different, but not incompatible, approaches: first, autonomy as the ideal that involves making decisions and actions one's own through rational reflection (Benn 1976; Dearden 1972); second, autonomy as an ideal of self-realization or self-fulfillment in which autonomy is valued as a means to achieve this end (Taylor 1979); and third, autonomy as a way of expressing moral integrity (Bettelheim 1960). Common to these approaches is that autonomy is regarded as a kind of character ideal or virtue. The differences between them might be regarded as differences of emphasis and focus rather than of rival conceptions of the ideal (Young 1986: 9–10).

The paradox of development and problems of identification

It might be thought wrong or even perverse to speak of development in connection with autonomy in long-term care when what we witness in long-term care is often the loss of capacity or the diminution of ability. After all, development means the progression from earlier to later stages of individual maturation, progress from the simpler to the more complex. To speak of a developmental perspective on autonomy may be relevant, but applying this view of autonomy to long-term care without major qualification surely romanticizes its harsh and unrelenting realities. Similarly, the process of identification seems to assume abilities that only infrequently occur in long-term care. If identification cannot be founded on the individual elder's own experience, it would seem to afford a ready platform for paternalism. The problem is that identification seems to imply a rather robust self-reflective ability that few elders needing long-term care actually possess. How can autonomy be useful ethically if abilities or capacities associated with it are routinely compromised or effaced in long-term care? If autonomy is truly a primary ethical concern in long-term care, then these reservations cannot be treated lightly.

Concern about the paradox of development and identification in the context of long-term care is related to fundamental questions about the underlying theory of the person or self that the concept of autonomy implies. Typically, such accounts are concerned more with ideal expressions of autonomy, with what the concept of autonomy means, than with elucidating actual manifestations of autonomy in the world of everyday experience. Such accounts are, nonetheless, relevant to the questions raised about development and identification, because they set the terms for the paradox. Critically discussing these theories helps us see why the focus on identification, as the core feature of autonomy, is consistent with and mutually supported by a developmental point of view. This discussion also provides a firm basis for the treatment of the phenomenology of action in the world of everyday life that comprises the next chapter.

Many recent treatments of the self view mental phenomena, such as beliefs, compulsions, desires, judgments, wishes, and so forth, as occurring on various levels. These so-called split-level theories of the self (Dworkin 1976, 1981, 1988; Frankfurt 1971; Jeffrey 1974; Neeley 1974; Young 1980a, 1980b), and accounts that do not use this exact terminology but still involve a remarkably similar hierarchical ordering of mental phenomena (Benn 1976; Bergmann 1977; Feinberg 1980; Taylor 1976), are increasingly taken to be important for explaining the problem of autonomous choice and the conditions under which it occurs (Friedman 1986). Autonomy as negative freedom seems oblivious to a range of common cases in which a person is a slave to convention and chooses in ways that derive uncritically from the social milieu (Benn 1976: 123). These cases press toward a more robust concept of autonomy that captures the root meaning of autonomy, namely, self-rule. An autonomous person in this fuller sense chooses not only in a way that is uncoerced, but also in a way that reflects his own goals, standards, ideals, or values. Beyond the requirement that an individual's choices be free of coercion and constraint, then, autonomy must involve some kind of reflection. The rub is that if the requirement for reflection is true in any stringent sense, than many of the conditions that engender the need for long-term care would also, by definition, rule out autonomy.

Many choices can be free in the sense of negative freedom, yet manifest mindless conformity to convention. Such cases are paradigm examples of choices that lack what might be termed *true autonomy*. As soon as this point is accepted, however, an important qualification is needed, because there are no clear limits to the extent to which the self can be thought of as biologically, psychologically, and sociologically determined. The self is determined by multiple developmental influences that combine to compose a sense of identity. If this is true, then it is unclear how a person could ever autonomously come to have values that are uniquely his own (Friedman 1986: 21). One well-known view holds that:

> If the autonomous man cannot adopt his motivations *do novo*, he can still judge them after the fact. The autonomous individual is still able to step back and formulate an attitude towards the factors that influence his behavior (Dworkin 1976: 24).

On this view, motivation becomes a person's own motivation as long as the person judges that she wants to be motivated as she is and as long as the judgment results from a process of critical reflection, a reflection that is free of manipulation, deception, or other constraint. In simplest terms, a person who approves of his motivations in this way *identifies* with them. This view has widespread support (Dworkin 1976: 25; Feinberg 1980: 8; Frankfurt 1971: 13;

Young 1980a: 37). The process involved is essentially one of self-reflection that judges one's first-order preferences according to a second or higher level of preferences, based on the highest principles available.

The problem with this account, as Marilyn Friedman rightly pointed out, is the special status that it accords critical reflection. Without critical reflection, there can be no true autonomy. This poses an important problem because if such a capacity is essential, then autonomy might prove to be rather rare, especially in long-term care. Critical reflection can confer autonomy in at least two different senses: first, the critically reflective self has a special ontological role in constituting the self as the true self; second, the process of critical reflection may involve the agent's identifying with her motivation. Such identification is sometimes taken to have ontological significance in that critical reflection is thought to be autonomy conferring just because it constitutes the 'higher,' 'real,' or 'true' self (Dworkin 1976: 24; Feinberg 1980: 19–20). Here, the liberal worry, discussed in Chapter 2, about covert metaphysical commitments in theories of positive autonomy seems to recur.

This problem is partly an artifact of the use of adjectives such as higher, real, or true in connection with the self. This language seems to imply an ontologically distinctive entity or component of self that comprises its essence. There is, however, no compelling reason to think that this need be the case, even though the talk of higher, real, or true selves is quite prominent in philosophic treatments of autonomy. In connection with specific cases or examples, such talk is usually understandable and not problematic. It seems natural and unobjectionable, for example, to speak about a true or higher self if the example involves a committed parent explaining why his family takes precedence over dedication to a favorite sport. Not traveling out of town to see a team play in deference to attending a child's school performance is comfortably expressed as an action and decision expressive of who the parent truly is or the higher values that the parent chooses to support as a parent.

Similarly, discussing one's religious convictions, arrived at after a long soul-searching examination, makes eminently good sense when expressed in terms of a notion of a higher or real self. However, to speak generally, especially in the context of philosophical analysis, of judging or evaluating one's first-order desires or preferences through a process of critical reflection in terms of a hierarchical apportionment of the self is misleading, given the tendency to reify the abstraction. The important point is that, although this mode of speaking is understandable and defensible in *specific analytic contexts*, problems occur when these terms are reified as elements or component parts of the self. When philosophers speak abstractly or universally about lower and higher levels, first-order and second-order motivations, and so on, no particular point of reference exists because the terminology is frequently detached from actual agency and actual autonomy. Although I have eschewed such approaches to autonomy, it makes sense to see whether identification, which is commonly expressed in just these kinds of abstract terms, can nonetheless be reattached to actual expressions of autonomy.

If autonomy primarily consisted in identification as understood by most split-level theorists, actions or choices would be autonomous only if the individual were capable of identifying with them in the sense that they would cohere with the true self. The source of autonomy, namely, the alleged true or higher self, however, is not itself necessarily autonomous to begin with. It is not clear that the *true* self is something that presupposes the operation of autonomy. As a result, the fact that a person identifies an element of her self as 'true' or 'identifies' with it does not assure that this part is really her true self or the basis of her identity. The relationship here is clearly contingent, and not logical. The fact that the relationship is not logical (or ontological) is a problem for split-level theories that appear to rely on such a certain priority. This need to have a fixed anchor is traceable to the rather abstract way that autonomy and agency are characterized in these treatments. Although the problem is difficult, it is tractable, especially in an account that adheres to actual autonomy.

The theoretical problem that split-level theorists must face is that critical reflection seems to be autonomy conferring, yet the highest principles that guide the reflective evaluation of lower-level choices and motivations, too, must be autonomy conferring (Friedman 1986: 29). Split-level accounts typically provide no adequate explanation of the way that autonomy could be conferred by a process whose highest principles themselves are not autonomously the agent's own. The split-level account of autonomy makes no provision for the realization of autonomy in respect to a person's highest values or principles. Nevertheless, this problem could be avoided if critical reflection did not have to be conceived as a purely top-down affair. If it must be top-down, then there is no room for autonomy at the top, and that is clearly paradoxical. The way out of this morass is to develop an account in which autonomy is conceived as a two-way process of integration involving a person's higher motivations, intermediate standards and values, and highest principles (Friedman 1986: 32).

One can usefully draw on an analogy with scientific explanation. Autonomy involves the process by which a person's covering principles, especially those at the highest level, are inducted from what they are supposed to cover, namely, lower-level choices or motivations. In other words, one builds up from experience, from one's actual choices and motivations, a sense of self that includes or is amenable to expression in terms of higher-level principles. This sense of self then serves as a normative principle for identification of subsequent experiences, choices, and so forth. Because this sense of self is a product of developmental influence, it is mainly an empirical product; it is not an ontological postulate. In other words, a person's higher values and principles, whatever ontological status they might have empirically, have to be subjected to assessment in terms of *actual* experience.

Although split-level theorists say that the higher or highest values and principles must be able to be judged rational by some special act or kind of critical reflection, they need not be actually reflected on; rather, the essential requirement is that they be lived and experienced as one's own, as cohering with the sense of one's developed self. How that might occur is an important psychological and phenomenological question, but it is not a matter to be settled by ethical theory. One relevant suggestion is that the life story and the narrative nature of life are far more important than usually appreciated by philosophers. The coherence at stake may not be ontological or logical at all, but aesthetic. If so, then standard conceptual commitments and styles of ethical analysis would need to be rather fundamentally rethought.

A self-concept becomes a personal concept only when it formatively shapes one's actions and is reciprocally reinforced by them. It is the product of an individual's developmental history. For this reason, attention to autonomy in long-term care necessarily involves attention to actual as opposed to ideal autonomy and to the phenomenology of the everyday life of elders. This focus necessarily constitutes a bottom-up form of assessment (Friedman 1986: 32). In this way, then, the problem of talking about development in the context of long-term care is rendered less perverse than it might first appear for elders in long-term care.

Identification is a process that occurs in the everyday experience of persons. One's sense of self is both formed and confirmed in the course of this experience in the world. As noted earlier, maturity is not an end-stage of a linear process of development, but rather a particular kind of development, one that involves self-mastery, achievement of effective competence in the world, as well as identification. To be an autonomous person in the world is to develop not toward some abstract ideal that, once attained, is then forever enacted, but as an integrative process of accommodating oneself to new circumstances and adapting those circumstances to one's unique structures of meaning. Identification thus precedes autonomy as independence (Bergmann 1977).

Even relatively abstract accounts like split-level accounts can be made to accommodate the concerns expressed earlier. In fact, the split-level approach encounters its unique set of problems mainly because it relies on an abstract hierarchical model of the self rather than on an integrated vision of the concrete person in the world. In a sense, the problems posed by development and identification are at least partly due to the metaphor underlying the discussion of choice, namely, to adapt Frost's phrase, two paths diverging in a wood. The metaphor of choice between alternatives obscures what is central in human action and choice, namely, uncertainty and the full range of background considerations that structure the perception of choices as open or viable. The path metaphor makes choice appear to be a matter of explicit options or alternatives made foresightfully, whereas this hardly captures the range of circumstances that are ethically important, particularly in long-term care, and it omits the uncertainty that characterizes lived experience.

Another metaphor might be more appropriate, namely, the metaphor of crossing a field of tall grass. Depending on where one entered the field and on one's interests, purposes, or needs, one might follow the natural gradient of the field, as in a leisurely stroll, or let it work against one, as an avid runner might do to build stamina. Certainly, the field might be crisscrossed with paths from previous travelers, but they will only be evident in the irregularities in the growing patterns of the grass, deviation from the perpendicular, but not as a smooth way. The influences of others and society will be patterns or tendencies, not causally determining forces. One might, of course, note these ways in advance and choose the one that afforded the least resistance, but the metaphor does not require that action and choice be so constrained. There is considerably more room for autonomy creatively and individually to make its own way across the field of experience. A person's action might be guided by the evident patterns marked out in the field, but they might also be guided by even more remote objectives like walking in the direction of flight of a grouse or a particular tree at the far end of the field.

The metaphor of the field of grass instead of the well-worn paths diverging in a wood metaphor is far more adequate for the purposes of understanding autonomy in long-term care. It is also more apt for understanding actual autonomy, but discussion of that point is beyond the limited objectives of this work. Its chief advantage is the way that it directs attention to a wider range of phenomena not normally thought of as relevant to the question of autonomous action and choice. In the next chapter, I show that, because actual autonomy involves being an agent in the everyday world, attention to certain structural features of that world can helpfully illuminate aspects of long-term care that might not normally be seen as features of autonomy.

Implications for long-term care

The foregoing discussion raises at least two important questions regarding long-term care. First, are the choices actually afforded individuals in long-term care the kind of choices that are meaningful or worth making? In other words, even when individuals are afforded choices, autonomy may not be significantly enhanced because the choices available may not be meaningful for the individuals involved. Ideally, choice that enhances autonomy is choice that is meaningful for individuals and allows them to express and develop their own individuality. If such is not the case, then the true sense of autonomy of persons is not enhanced.

Consider, for example, the kinds of choices that are typically afforded individuals in nursing homes. There are choices regarding limited outings, the use of special services such as hairdressing, or participation in structured social and recreational activities such as bingo. No matter how extensive this list of choices is, one can ask whether the choices are meaningful for the individuals. Does the list include choices that preserve and enhance the elders' individuality and identity, such as choosing when and what to eat, or do they have permission to choose to ask for help or to refuse help from staff? If it is the case that the actual choices afforded to individuals in nursing homes are not seen by those individuals as meaningful, but that other choices that are not made available are seen as meaningful, then serious questions arise regarding how autonomy is being respected in these circumstances. This suggests that caregivers and managers must attend more thoroughly to the question of the meaningfulness of the choices actually afforded elders under their care.

Being able to identify with one's choices is a prerequisite for true autonomy. There are choices which individuals can be forced to make that negate the integrity and self-worth of the person. In the movie *Sophie's Choice*, a Jewish woman was made to choose either her son or daughter for extermination on entry into a Nazi concentration camp. Although she did choose, her choice was not one with which she could rationally or sanely identify. Hence, that choice haunts her throughout life. It is a surd or irrational element in her life that distorts her ability to love and function as a mature person. Similar, though less dramatic, kinds of choices are also confronted by elders or families with disabled elders requiring long-term care.

The 75-year-old woman whose own health is deteriorating must make choices regarding the care of her 78-year-old husband who has suffered a stroke and is now bedridden. Similarly, the husband must choose institutionalization or watch as his wife is consumed by caring for him. The family of such a couple also faces equally difficult choices. Do they take the couple into their households for care? Do they break up the couple and arrange for different care for each of their parents? Are the alternatives available in long-term care meaningful for elders? Can they identify with the alternatives? Sometimes, the cost to self for the elder in agreeing to move in with children is too great, not because the elder prizes independence, but because the elder cannot identify with a choice that imposes burdens on children and means the loss of friends or familiar surroundings.

The psychological consequence of this point is evident everywhere in long-term care. As Bergmann has pointed out, nonidentification characteristically carries with it a sense of passivity: 'Once the subject structures his experience in a certain way, he has to feel passive, but the sense of passivity in turn reinforces nonidentification: the self that is overwhelmed at every moment withdraws still further' (1977: 48). Thus, the withdrawal and generalized depression that one often sees in institutionalized elders may be traced to the existentially tragic choices that elders are forced to make or to endure. Recognizing this point is clinically helpful, even if the situation of tragic choice generally defies solution by society.

If altering one's identifications is sometimes too formidable a task or requires too long term a solution, then we should look elsewhere to address the sequelae of tragic choice. If we are serious about enhancing the autonomy of elders in long-term care, but are unable to modify social and institutional patterns of care, then we must turn specifically to the ways that long-term care is locally implemented and introduce modifications that hold the promise of at least remedially addressing the issue of respect for persons. This is, in effect, the second question that autonomy as identification poses for long-term care.

If the actual exercise of choice is typically only a small part of our lives, then questions about the style of life and the structure and organization of long-term care assume importance. In other words, is the style of life available in long-term care meaningful for elders? Is the life available in long-term care something with which the elder can identify, that is, not through explicit choice but passively and reflexively? Raising this question suggests that a radically different metaphor of autonomy in long-term care is required (Agich 1995a). In this new picture, there are no walls and everything is open. There are not, as in the traditional view, decision-making nodes along a narrow path that diverges at certain points: the decision to institutionalize or to accept skilled-level care. Instead, autonomy is always present, though sometimes hidden from view as individuals go about their daily lives. Every step and every move we make could have been different, though it seldom seems to be.

We are carried forward in our lives by a constant and monotonous exercise of choice of which we are all but oblivious. Choice does not hover only between two alternatives; there is rarely just a simple fork, a stark either/or; rather, at every step, we could have moved in countless possible directions whether we realize it or not (Bergmann 1977: 77). That is why I insisted earlier that the proper understanding of autonomy involves appreciating how individuals are interconnected and determined by historical and social factors. Human growth and development are not simply a procession of stages through which we pass to become adult, independent decision makers, but a dynamic adaptation and encounter with the world that persists throughout our lives. Autonomy is the essential spontaneity that defines human personhood and is ever present. The acquisition habits of action and thought are as much socially derived as they are individually and uniquely determined, but they are adopted spontaneously through effortful action by each individual. Thus, we need to pay more attention to the psychosocial correlates of autonomy and to the arrangements that either foster or thwart the development and expression of individuality and personhood.

Taking identification seriously requires us to face a particularly problematic question. As discussed in Chapter 3, nursing homes are remarkably heterogeneous and complex social and cultural systems. Hence, they are fraught with potential conflicts. It is simply not reasonable to expect that ethnic or racial stereotypes that developed over a lifetime will disappear as one enters a nursing home as a resident or staff member (Foldes 1990: 24). These markers of identity do not magically fade away when people become old and sick, so the question arises: what if the central values and beliefs of elders are discriminatory, mean, or selfish?

The requirements of autonomy as independence certainly support individuals manifesting and maintaining attitudes and beliefs that are not ethically defensible, but only as long as those attitudes and beliefs do not infringe on the rights of others. Concern and respect for the rights of others are ethically required. Liberal principles clearly support this assertion, but also do not help much in understanding the ethical demands that autonomy places on a particular person. It is inadequate to acknowledge that someone is truly a bigot and let matters rest there. Actual autonomy requires appeal to the primary sense of responsibility that essentially characterizes what it means to be an autonomous agent. Concern and respect for others are not optional for the truly autonomous self; they are basic obligations, because they support the very conditions necessary for a formed self.

Despite the complex historical, institutional, and social character of our understandings of disease and health (Agich 1983a; Caplan, Engelhardt, and McCartney 1981; Twaddle 1979), it is clear that there is a striking divergence between contemporary acute-oriented concepts of disease and chronic-oriented concepts. In their analysis of unpublished data from the Health Interview Survey the National Nursing Home Study, L.H. Butler and P.W. Newacheck found that almost the entire decline in health associated with increasing age is accounted for by chronic rather than acute conditions (1981). Similarly, as L. Cluff has noted with regard to chronic disease, acute or episodic care alone is inadequate. The expectation and goal of care should not be the elimination of disease, which by definition in chronic conditions is not possible, but rather maintenance of function (1981).

Given that elders seem more likely than younger persons to experience functional disabilities as the result of chronic illnesses (Fredman and Haynes 1985), services should be available that adequately meet these needs. *Functional disability* points to the degree to which an illness or impairment interferes with meaningful daily living. These are often measured in empirical studies by the number of days lost from housework, school, work, or days spent in bed (Butler and Newacheck 1981). The concept of functional ability measures the impact of an illness or impairment on the individual and on the individual's ability to engage and interact in the social world, instead of the presence or absence of disease. Indeed, some have noted that 'the loss or impairment of the ability to perform such basic daily functions as shopping or bathing strikes at what the elderly value most – independent living' (Pegels 1981: 5). Independent living here does not mean autonomy conceived as independence, but autonomy as identification. It means the kind of life that coheres with the elder's own sense of self. The ability to perform normal functions of daily living is best understood in terms of the individual's basic sense of self-worth, how the elder identifies herself. One challenge for institutional long-term care is to develop supportive substitutes for the activities that elders value, but can no longer perform.

Loss of function is an important concern is documented in the research that finds no association in the minds of elders between health and the presence of chronic illness or disability (Ferraro 1980; Fillenbaum 1979). In some studies, 68 percent of noninstitutionalized elders report their health as excellent or good, despite the fact that 85 percent have at least one chronic illness and 47 percent have some functional disability (Filner and Williams 1979; Kovar 1977). In 1994–5, 52.5 percent of the older population reported that they have at least one disability, but only 14 percent reported difficulty in carrying out activities of daily living (Administration on Aging 2000). Many individuals experience themselves as healthy if they maintain functional ability even in the face of chronic disease. The account of autonomy just offered helps to explain why this is so.

Maintaining a sense of autonomous well-being is consistent with dependencies on medication or professional care if those dependencies help to maintain a more basic sense of functional integrity in those areas of life that individuals value. Dependencies as such do not conflict with autonomy if individuals can still maintain a sufficiently adequate range of identifications to sustain their personal sense of integrity and worth.

These observations help to explain why focusing on acute illness and episodic interventions has such dramatic implications for the concept of autonomy in long-term care. Given an acute disease-driven model of health care, specific decisions such as those regarding institutionalization, skilled nursing care, withholding or withdrawing technological life supports naturally become prominent. Correlatively, worries about infringement of individuals' fundamental rights naturally arise and support the belief that autonomy is properly and exclusively to be conceived as independence and noninterference. In such a view, what seems less pressing, even insignificant, are the mundane aspects of long-term care. Attention to everyday ethics (Kane and Caplan 1990), however, is a necessary component of any serious and sustained treatment of actual autonomy in long-term care.

Robert Kastenbaum has correctly noted that we often see the clinical ambience minus the clinical benefits. The person who is a patient only temporarily can adjust to the unfamiliar and unlovely hospital routines knowing that this is only an interlude. Some comfort and individuality is sacrificed; however, in fair return the person receives state-of-the-art medical and nursing care. By contrast, the geriatric milieu is a long-term or permanent arrangement for many people, and the clinical ambience is not counterbalanced by superb care. Perhaps the most infuriating note from the standpoint of the patient is the attitude that 'this is all for your own good.' It is not – and everybody knows it (1983: 11).

Although nursing dominates the nursing home, registered nurses are seldom regularly seen by residents. Instead, licensed practical nurses (LPNs) and certified nursing assistants (CNAs) provide most care. A bitter irony for most institutionalized elders is that the disruptive move to the nursing home is predicated on their having medical needs that require around-the-clock care, when they typically seldom have contact with a physician or nurse after their admission (Kane 1990: 12).

Kastenbaum argues that the necessary goal for the clinical milieu is less a matter of specific medical or nursing interventions than 'making the world right again' (1983: 12–15). Frail and impaired older persons experience many sorrows, losses, fears, and frustrations in addition to physical ailments and disabilities. A truly therapeutic environment would certainly provide treatments that ameliorate discomfort and help individuals maintain a level of integrated functioning, but, more importantly, would also attend to the everyday routine and quality of experience of the residents. The safest generalization one can make regarding the experience of the nursing home is that it is boring (Kane 1990: 17). There are long stretches in which elders have nothing to look forward to except the next meal. No wonder, then, that institutionalized elders have been found to engage in activities that might seem to casual observers to be relatively bizarre and apparently meaningless, such as watching cars (Gubrium 1975: 180–4). This behavior, however, is far from passive, since it represents an engaged and autonomous activity of elders who have serious functional limitations. It is an example of an elder engaging in the social world of everyday life that is severely restricted by physical and environmental factors. As Timothy Diamond reported, based on his own participant observation:

I came to change my image of nursing home life as a static enterprise. It is not sitting in a chair 'doing nothing.' Rather than being passive, it is always a process. Each person is situated in a overall turbulent path. Each person sits in a chair or lies in a bed, often appearing motionless, but is moving and being moved, however silently, through the society. (1986: 1289)

Talking, walking, and watching were actually quite important activities for elders at Murray Manor, the institution where Diamond did his primary observations. They represented various ways that elders who appeared to be 'just sitting around' were actually engaged in a personally meaningful activity. When observed to be just sitting, both elders and staff reported nervousness and anxiety; it was associated with unnecessary requests for help or requests for assistance in toileting that produced no urine or stool. The psychological and social dynamic of these requests raises the questions 'What were the elders seeking? What were they trying to do? What are some of the relevant conditions of actual autonomy in long-term care?'

The consequence of these points is that an ethic of long-term care must attend to what Hans Selye termed the *syndrome of just being sick* (1956: 79), namely, that things are just *not right*. Besides specific disabilities and pains, disabled elders sense the world has gone awry; they experience a pervasive sense of loss or what might simply be termed *existential despair*. Kastenbaum argues that the *just being sick* syndrome can be countered effectively only by a milieu that accentuates the positive, a milieu that develops a systematic and encompassing framework of positive expectations on the part of everyone involved. Clarifying the components of such a milieu would be one way to manifest concern for autonomy. To do that, however, requires the concept of autonomy to be refurbished in ways that show how actual autonomy is manifest in the social world of everyday life.

Summary

In this chapter, we have discussed result-oriented and action-oriented or agent-oriented ethical theories and argued that the latter afford a more adequate basis for conceptualizing autonomy. Unfortunately, insofar as they rely on an abstract rather than a concrete view of human persons, even action-oriented or agent-oriented theories do not carry us far enough. Reliance on abstract views of action and choice is problematic, because it reduces the complex reality of autonomy in health care to the idealization of a competent, rational free agent. Actually, such idealizations are infrequently present in long-term care. A wide chasm exists between ideal competence and actual incompetence.

Central to the concept of actual autonomy is the view that identification precedes autonomy and, indeed, is a more primary phenomenon in terms of which autonomy as choice should be analyzed. Identification is a common-enough theme in recent philosophical treatments of autonomy. We have seen how adhering to actual autonomy solves certain theoretical problems associated with typical split-level approaches. The main point to draw from this discussion is that what autonomy actually means in the everyday world of long-term care is likely to exceed by a rather long margin the usual range of philosophical analysis that focuses on abstract cases and problems.

Respecting the autonomy of persons in long-term care entails a commitment to identifying and establishing the concrete conditions that encourage individuals to face adversity and threats to self that are the inevitable result of the chronic illnesses and functional deteriorations that bring elders to long-term care in the first place. Respecting autonomy requires attending to those things that are truly and significantly meaningful and important for elders. This means that elders must be treated as individuals, as unique persons with identifiable personal histories and a rich store of experiences and memories. When such identifications are difficult to assess, as in cases of severe memory or cognitive impairments, elders sometimes respond, albeit minimally and in deficient ways, to direct contact with caregivers and others. Long-term care can provide positive messages and hope, even in the face of serious impairment. Hope does not mean recovery, however, as is usually assumed in the medical context; instead, hope refers to the prospect of meaningful experience with others at those times when one most needs comfort and companionship. The natural tendency of long-term care is to distort self-perception and to deny the social functioning of elders. The phenomenological framework for understanding autonomy that we consider in the next chapter is meant to provide a framework for improving our sensitivity to expressions of actual autonomy in long-term care and, ultimately, to improve the milieu of long-term care itself.

5

A phenomenological view of actual autonomy

Philosophical treatments of autonomy typically rely on idealized examples that are far removed from the ordinary actions that make up everyday experience. The ethical problems associated with long-term care, however, extend far beyond these examples into a domain of experience that makes up everyday life. *Actual autonomy* is manifested not in such rarified examples, but in the everyday actions in the shared world of social life. The features of actual autonomy are to be found not in distinctive decision-making nodes, but in the interstitial features of everyday life (Agich 1995a). Once we appreciate the interdependent character of being an autonomous agent in the world, the implications of autonomy for long-term care can be discussed without being restricted to the ideals of independence and noninterference. This chapter develops some general features of the social world and what it means to be a person existing in that world. Autonomy is seen as a core feature of persons in this view, but persons are seen as essentially connected with, rather than isolated from, others and the world. Four exemplary aspects of the phenomenology of the social existence of persons are particularly relevant to autonomy in long-term care: the spatial, temporal, communicative, and affective dimensions. Implications for long-term care are drawn for each of these dimensions of social action. This discussion thus provides a basic framework for reassessing and reconceptualizing the problems associated with autonomy in long-term care.

Sociality and the world of everyday life

We have discussed the liberal concept of autonomy and sketched a set of considerations supporting a view of actual autonomy involving identifications. The thrust of this analysis is that persons are interdependent; as agents, they exist in the social world of everyday life and their autonomy emerges and has its terminus therein. These considerations can be taken in either of two directions: communitarianism or a phenomenological account of actual autonomy. The first well-known approach views sociality as a guide to a distinctive ethic, an ethic that stresses human relationships, commitment, and tradition as central values. Sociality elevates the community over the individual. Autonomy as an ideal of the isolated, abstract decision maker obviously has no place in such a scheme. As a general theory of human nature that denies the importance of shared commitments, the liberal view of autonomy is surely suspect, but one need not reject this view entirely. As a political doctrine according to which government should treat persons as free individuals, that is, apart from status and ascription, liberal theory is definitely worth saving. Community and tradition provide no unassailable values. Of course, the critics of liberalism are correct in pointing out its deficiencies as an ethical theory. These deficiencies, however, do not invalidate its importance within the compass of politics and public life. Thus, distinguishing the liberal view of autonomy as a theory of human nature and a theory of politics is crucial. One can preserve the distinctive contribution of liberal thought to modern culture and society, namely, its protection of individuals from the intrusive power of the state and other individuals and enhancement of the status of persons, while at the same time acknowledging that this view presents at best a truncated understanding of the nature of persons, moral obligation, and ethics.

Critics of liberalism, however, point out that when autonomy is taken in its libertarian form, any meaningful sense of community or tradition, which they regard as foundational for morality, is inevitably lost, because apparently anything that a free individual desires or prefers and can freely choose becomes morally acceptable for a liberal. Such a view is ultimately incoherent and indefensible. That it has any credibility whatever attests to the degree to which the legal understanding of rights and the political understanding of autonomy infuse contemporary thought to the exclusion of other considerations. Communitarians, unfortunately, propose to address these problems globally by substituting a focus on community and tradition for the liberal ideal of autonomous free choice. Such a substitution, however, rejects the core tenet of liberalism, namely, that liberty is a central value in politics and, instead, proposes a philosophical anthropology in which community is central. This approach denatures the ethical into the political and attempts to resolve political and ethical problems by appealing to a substantive philosophical anthropology or metaphysics that is hardly universal. These problems lead us to consider a second approach to sociality, one that brackets or methodologically sets aside these typical understandings of autonomy in order to examine autonomy's actual manifestation in the everyday world of experience.

On this second view, sociality is an essential feature of being a person. This is a descriptive, phenomenological claim about human existence and not a metaphysical claim as offered by the communitarian. As such, it does not establish an ethic, but provides a framework for articulating an ethic of autonomy and long-term care. This claim has no explanatory force in itself. In this approach, a description of the social nature of personal autonomy is offered. No normative ethical claims are directly made with respect to sociality as a feature of personal autonomy, but some main ways that autonomy is manifested in the common social world are described. These features collectively provide a framework for thinking about autonomy and long-term care. Drawing out the implications for an ethics of long-term care, however, is not a task directly undertaken in this work.

Instead, we focus our understanding on the ways that the social world provides the background or framework against which any adequate theory of autonomy in long-term care will ultimately need to be measured. In typical discussions of autonomy, sociality is left in the background and does not receive explicit attention. It provides a stage upon which the foreground discussion of autonomy arises. The phenomenological treatment of actual autonomy directs attention to these background features of sociality that make personal autonomy possible. Sociality and the social world of everyday life provide the scaffolding or framework for autonomy. The social world thus gives us the basic source of meaning for personal autonomy in all its forms. Even the most abstract philosophical articulations of autonomy are based on the everyday features of autonomous action in the world. Throwing light on this background will allow us to see how actual autonomy functions in the everyday world.

The everyday world is an important concept for gauging actual autonomy, because whatever autonomy actually involves, its locus and referent are the world of everyday life. The commonsense or everyday world provides the setting for judging the adequacy of any ethics. It does so because the everyday world is a practical world of doing. It forms what Alfred Schutz (1971a: 226–9, 341–4) has termed the *paramount reality* within which our lives are lived and which provides the reality or content that all practical reflection seeks to clarify. This world is a historical world in which human beings come into existence and acquire their standing as agents or persons. It is the place wherein lives are lived, actions undertaken, and choices made. It is important to emphasize that the term *world of everyday life* refers to a zone of experience that is not limited. Even though the term might be mistaken to imply only the ordinary, routine, or common aspects of existence from which the celebrated, dramatic, or rare has been excluded, everyday life includes surprises and the unexpected. The feature that defines the world of everyday life is not so much its familiarity, though it certainly is familiar, as the fact that it is the taken-for-granted place in which we act, experience, and live our lives. The *everyday world* thus refers to that omnipresent background for our actions. Other realities or *finite provinces of meaning* (Schutz 1971a: 207–59, 340–7) such as imagined worlds can have rich articulations, but they are not where we *live* or share a world of life and work with others. The everyday life world is the place where we interact as agents with each other and things. It is the place where autonomy actually dwells and where we must look if we want to observe autonomy in action. As Egon Bittner has pointed out, 'It is impossible to overestimate the *centrality of the subject* for the phenomenal constitution of this world of everyday life' (1973: 119–20).

That is why, if we are to fully understand the manifold expressions of autonomy, we need to look to the world of everyday life.

The everyday commonsense world is the world of everyday life in which we carry out our day-to-day affairs. In this world we operate on the basis of typical or taken-for-granted ways of understanding and doing things. For example, in cooking a meal we take for granted the foods we prepare based on habitual preference. We are not usually reflectively concerned with where the food came from, how the electricity or gas used to cook the food was produced and delivered to us, or whether food producers and utilities producers are profiting. Instead, we are attentive to what immediately needs to be done: making sure the skillet is hot enough, finding the oil, scrambling the egg, and so on. These actions are routinized as part of the cooking skills we possess. Precisely because such activities are routinized and the meanings of things in the world are typified, the world of everyday life conceals its internal complexity from us. We do not know how we came to prefer scrambled to over-easy eggs or how we developed our technique in breaking the eggs. We engage and live in our activities and give our full attention to the objects or objectives of our actions within the world without reflecting on our activities and the source of meaning. We are typically engaged in the world, simply busy with the many concerns and activities that make up our lives.

To call these activities routine signifies that they are both commonplace and to a great extent automatic or habitual. The most routine and regular of our activities – indeed, activities that are not so much active as automatic – are the result of developmental achievements and efforts in the reflexive interaction of the person as agent with the world. Importantly, the fully developed person, who is the ideal of liberal thought, is capable of rational decision making precisely because, as an embodied and socially formed self, he is able to rely unthinkingly on acquired habits and skills. Consider, for example, the effort necessary for an adult to regain the ability to walk after an incapacitating injury. What is so easy, so ordinary, so automatic before the injury becomes, for the individual needing rehabilitation, a matter of effort and striving. Each step requires a conscious exercise of the will that confronts a recalcitrant body. The need for effort and striving, basic elements of what autonomy developmentally involves, is everywhere evident in long-term care as elders are forced by their frailties and cognitive and physical incapacities to adapt and adjust themselves to the world.

As agents, we function in the everyday world precisely on the basis of abilities, habits, and skills acquired historically. We rely on typifications that embody our unique personal, familial, and cultural values and beliefs that suffuse the things of the world and our experiences with meaning. Each person enacts his unique developmental history in the everyday world. The underlying view of the person as an agent in the everyday world involves the recognition that human experience, despite the modern tendency to separate body and mind, is essentially embodied (Johnson 1987; Merleau-Ponty 1962, 1967). Actual autonomy is thus to be found not in the mental processes of deliberation and choice, but primarily in embodied action. To be a person is to have a future that is in a basic sense open, but always limited by our past and present abilities and limitations.

Underlying these limitations is our finitude and the inevitability of death that forms the backdrop of the everyday world. When things fail to function, when things do not go right in the ordinary course of everyday experience, then we become aware, though often only inchoately, of our nature as finite and embodied persons. Alfred Schutz pointed out that the *fundamental anxiety* (1971a: 226–9) about our finitude is at the root of our everyday experience. This anxiety propels our actions in the everyday world, but our routine experience overlooks this anxiety as we lose ourselves in our busy-ness with the things and projects of our world. Illness is the common paradigm type of experience in which the possibility of a fundamental disruption between the self and existence in the world is experienced. In illness we universally come to awareness of the limits of our existence and mastery of the world. We experience our own selves, our bodies, as part of the world of things that break down. In the natural world, we experience ourselves as biological beings whose coming to be and living are framed by the inevitability of our passing away. We act, experience, and live in the world as embodied and finite creatures whose existence is always perilous.

To be autonomous thus necessarily involves an essential adhesion to the everyday world. Hence, to be free cannot, except on the basis of a convenient abstraction, mean that one is isolated and independently able to exercise rational decisions. Rather, actual autonomy involves the use of elements or features of one's own self that are precarious and presently not completely free, precisely because they involve aspects of self that are embodied *automatically* as acquired habits or skills.

General features of the social nature of persons

To function as an agent in the world requires that individuals have a broad set of abilities or skills, a *stock of knowledge at hand*, that is acquired through habituation (Schutz 1970: 75–102, 133–62). The processes whereby acquisition of basic skills necessary for agency occurs provide the empirical basis for the view of parentalism discussed in Chapter 2 and it underlies the developmental view of autonomy discussed in Chapter 4. The stock of knowledge at hand is made up of a variety of abilities that developed over time and are sedimented often in a complexly interdependent or hierarchical fashion. It provides the foundation for our ability to act in the world. To be an individual agent capable of independent action in the social world thus requires relationships with others – others who necessarily figure in the development and sustenance of the abilities that allow an individual to be free. This point cannot be overstressed.

The fundamental meaning of the autonomy of a person is thus bound up with that person's relationships with others: relationships with those who fostered the acquisition of basic motor and communication skills as well as with those individuals who provided reinforcement and further development of skills throughout life. Acquisition of skills and abilities to negotiate the world is an essential prerequisite for the development of a sense of self and mature personhood. To be an autonomous agent, one needs prior relationships in which the fundamental processes of human growth and development can occur (Bowlby 1969, 1973, 1980; Spitz 1965). Far from being isolated centers of independent decision making or action, human persons are agents in the everyday world precisely insofar as they are sustained by a complex web of interconnections and relationships with both past and present others. The concrete reality of autonomy, therefore, bears little or no resemblance to the abstract picture provided by the liberal theory.

In order to function at all as agents in the world of everyday life, we regularly take a number of things for granted. We engage in actions and experience the world on the basis of *typifications*. Typifications provide frames through which events are experienced and made meaningful to us. By organizing expectations, they introduce a flexible ordering of experience. As a corollary, typifications elaborate an understanding that allows us to relate to otherwise unconnected experiences or events. For example, an institutionalized elder may experience any caregiver as nurse, a concept that indicates a generalized set of expectations regarding competence, knowledge, and function as well as expectations about the care that will be provided. Caregiving staff members similarly typify elders in terms of disease categories or as *feeders*, namely, those who need help eating. These terms denote rather heterogeneous classes that are nonetheless meaningfully associated in everyday experience. Such associations serve as practical guides to action by suggesting responses and by structuring further expectations. Besides guiding action and organizing experience, typifications also have a profound rhetorical function, that is, they persuade and convince others about the proper interpretation of one's own and others' acts (Gubrium and Buckholdt 1977: 58–62). Typifications work effectively because they express or involve shared social understandings.

The function of typifications is to collectively provide the means by which the everyday world is negotiated. *Negotiation* means to accommodate, accomplish, or cope with something, as in 'negotiating a sharp curve' in driving an automobile, and 'to arrange or settle by conferring or discussing with others' as when one negotiates a contract. Both aspects of the term are at work in the world of everyday experience as individuals interact with the world and each other. The everyday world involves the suspension of doubt in the possibility that things might be otherwise than they appear. Doubt and disbelief, however, are intrinsic to human freedom, yet the attitude of life in the everyday world involves a basic trust that takes for granted that things are functioning as they are supposed to. As a result, we engage unreflectively in activities in the everyday world until the taken-for-granted ways of doing things fail. The experience of failures, problems, difficulties, and obstacles gives pause to our engaged activity and occasions reflection. These failures force us to evaluate our situation, which involves stepping back from the world. Such disengagement is a prerequisite for reevaluation and choice and is a basic feature of freedom that philosophers usually treat as a high-order cognitive function. To require that autonomy involve such higher order functioning, however, is misleading. To be an autonomous agent first and foremost means that the world as an object of experience is held in dynamic relationship by the intentional nature of consciousness itself. It is this dynamic power that is at the basis of the spontaneity that comprises autonomy in its most basic form. Such a power underlies the capability of trying to (creatively) alter that involvement, an ability that often appears to be called forth by circumstances outside our control. Ironically, one common assumption of the traditional liberal view is that autonomy consists in the absence of obstacles when actual autonomy awakens precisely when occlusions are encountered in daily living.

Frithjof Bergmann argued that the traditional concept of autonomy wrongly assumes both an absence of relationship and an absence of obstacles to choice or desire (1977: 41–53). The liberal view simply assumes that desire should hold sway no matter what. Everything, including social or ethical norms, historical and cultural circumstances, interpersonal relationships, or a number of other contingencies, must be swept aside as autonomy expresses itself in the world. True freedom is freedom without opposition. This view is fundamentally mistaken. When there are no obstacles, failures, problems, or difficulties, one is simply busy, and so unreflectively bonded in habituated ways of involvement with the world and things. In these circumstances, autonomy is submerged. To be sure, only when routines break down, when normal expectations are frustrated, and when relationships come undone do reflection and conscious exercise of choice really enter. Only an abstract account would regard the fecund experiences between the nodes of conflict or choice as nonfreedom. Of course, if one uncritically assumes that the person is primarily a rational decision maker and rationality is understood in intellectual terms, then the idea of an autonomous person acting unreflectively would surely seem strange. The strangeness of this picture depends upon the strong and unexamined association of rationality and freedom.

Despite the many kinds of frustration in our everyday experience of the world, we are usually able to attend sufficiently to practicalities so that we manage. For example, confusion, distraction, feeling down, forgetfulness, and myriad other symptomatic alterations in consciousness associated with ill-ness deflect and distort the attention our everyday engagement in the world seems to demand. Even normal routinized activities become burdensome and difficult when illness or disability occurs, because our basic bodily standing, our upright orientation in the world, is affected (Straus 1963: 137–65). So-called coping strategies usually involve utilizing or developing techniques to ameliorate the disengagement from the everyday world that illness or other experiences associated with daily living foist on us. Because many of these dislocations are themselves fairly routine and expected, we possess various techniques for adapting or coping.

The need to cope points out how central the social world of everyday life is to our very existence as human persons. We cope and adapt because we must get on with things, because we must engage in the world at hand. Reflection can be fruitfully regarded as the intellectual corollary of the wide range of adapting and coping behaviors that are routinely exhibited in daily life. It is the intellectual or cognitive expression of autonomy that presupposes the ability to disengage from involvement with, indeed bondage to, things in the everyday world. Reflection, however, occurs in the everyday world precisely when one's usual habits of thought or patterns of behavior are disrupted by either external or internal factors. What philosophers call *reflection* is primarily a disengaged, intellectual activity. It is a type of a much more common and variegated psychological process that is an essential feature of all human life. It is manifested in the everyday world in problem solving and mundane, taken-for-granted decision making about rather ordinary and unremarkable matters. To be autonomous, then, does not mean that one must be free to choose in a Sartrean vacuum, as it were, but to act in the midst of things and at the behest of things and events.

Explicit, self-aware reflection (as well as conscious or explicit choice) emerges from our daily interaction with the world and others. Infants are not born autonomous, but acquire freedom in the world as they develop skills and abil-ities that allow them to deal competently with the world (Haworth 1986). Hence, the phenomenological reality of human autonomy consists in its ad-herence to the world. Adherence is an important concept. By adherence, I mean to suggest a relationship much like that of a plant enrooted in the earth. The earth does not hold it fast, but rather the plant, through its root structure, holds itself fast to the earth and draws nutrients therefrom. Similarly, the hu-man person is bound to the world by the very nature of its existence and so the connection with the world is not one of bondage or enslavement, but of active attachment. Autonomous relations of human persons with the world and with one another are misconstrued in any model that exclusively focuses on independence or negative freedom. To properly understand the nature of autonomy, then, it is necessary to take seriously the nature of human persons in their concrete involvement in the social world.

A significant feature of the social world of everyday life is that it assumes common or shared culture (Garfinkel 1962). This common culture provides the taken-for-granted grounds for understanding and acting that make the everyday world a common or shared public space. This world is public in the sense that it is defined in terms of objective or clock time that makes common schedules possible (Zerubavel 1981). Objective extension or space provides a reference that defines your there and my here and it orders our expectation of the way things happen in the world, namely, sequentially or in joint occurrence and interaction. Sociologists have pointed out that the commonality of the social world involves shared beliefs and values that in a general way define what we experience as normal or usual.

This observation is relevant for ethics since all practical reasoning arises from asking the question 'What am I to do?' Asking that question, of course, has point only when some reason has presented itself or been presented to the agent for doing something other than what is normal or typical. Reasons for acting are good, or are effective in guiding action when they function as causes. A cause is always something that makes a difference to an outcome. In human action, the processes and procedures for which reasons for action make a causal difference are primarily those that bite into the everyday world and alter or engage its routine. The concept of the normal day, month, year, and so on is of the first importance in understanding human action and reasoning about action in any culture. Philosophers have unfortunately shown remarkably little interest in the mundane, even though the structure of everyday normality provides the most basic framework for understanding human action.

Acting in accordance with the structures of the everyday world does not require that the agent be able to articulate rational reasons for acting, except in certain specific circumstances in which those structures have been put in question. Mundane necessities, such as eating at prescribed times, in prescribed company, occur without anyone having to give reasons for them. In similar fashion, work or other activities follows a routine pattern, if not formal schedule. Rituals occupy parts of the routinized day and reinforce the habits of structured activity. Even play and casual pursuits have their own structure and own place within the larger structures of the everyday world (MacIntyre 1988: 24–5; Zerubavel 1981).

Acting for specific rational reasons is usually the exception. In normal circumstances, rational action is intelligible only in terms of and against the background structures of everyday social normality. Action that departs from the background social expectations and norms usually requires that one have and be able to give reasons, typically for exemption from the tacitly accepted standards. What counts as an adequate or good reason for action is therefore first and foremost a reason good enough for doing something other than that which normality prescribes. The mark of a good reason is not intellectual or formal, but pragmatic rationality, namely, what works or what is accepted. Alasdair MacIntyre pointed out:

... when a reason is judged to outweigh the requirements of the customary structure, there is in the background the possibility of a not-yet formulated judgment of some kind as to how good the reasons are for doing what the customary structure prescribes. And so reasoning which justifies particular requirements of that structure may emerge from the reasoning which puts it in question. But only in this secondary way do agents find reasons for doing what is normally prescribed. (1988: 25)

In point of fact, the structures of everyday normality serve primarily to make it unnecessary for most people most of the time to provide explanations for what they are doing or are about to do. Because most of what we do conforms to these general norms of everyday life, we are relieved of what would otherwise be an intolerable burden. This, of course, does not mean that the structures of the everyday world are transparent to understanding, but that for the agents involved they are more like the air we breathe, essential, yet completely unremarkable.

The agent in the everyday world is thus an essentially dependent entity, dependent on a socially derived stock-of-knowledge at hand and a repertoire of abilities and skills that comprise the background against which individual difference is manifested. In many respects, the focus on autonomy in ethics is best interpreted as recognition of, or, indeed, insistence on, the importance of a sense of self, of individuality as a core concept for ethics, rather than as a claim for complete independence. That explains, in part, why many find the concept of autonomy to be a touchstone in ethics and medical ethics. The crucial issue is whether autonomy as it is theoretically understood is sufficiently rich to endow autonomy with the substance and breadth it requires if it is to play the central role assigned to it in ethics. My earlier discussion of the liberal theory of autonomy was motivated by the belief that the typical expressivist account provides an inadequate or thin view of personhood, a view that is too narrow to support and sustain significant inquiry into the ethics of long-term care. A theory of autonomy that provides a concrete view of persons must be one that is sensitive to the social nature of personhood and to the complex conditions that actually support the unique identity of those individuals needing long-term care.

Adaptation to the social dislocation and physical disability that usually precipitates the need for long-term care occurs within the social world and needs to be understood against this backdrop. It is thus a fundamental mistake to regard individuals, even severely confused, withdrawn, or psychotic individuals, as somehow completely apart from the social world. Their involvement may be pathological and their functioning may be deviant, precarious, or marginal, but insofar as such individuals can be regarded as human persons in any minimal sense, they, too, occupy the shared world of everyday life.

Perhaps the best example of this point is autism. Gerhard Bosch noted that one of the most striking features of autistic life consists in what he called *positive peculiarities*, which define what it means to be autistic:

Once one has trained oneself to see these 'positive peculiarities' of autistic children, it will be clear that they are extraordinarily attached to certain family situations, to being looked after by a certain person, and to a rigidly followed daily routine within which tenderness, such as a going-to-bed ritual with a good-night kiss and certain morning greetings, all have their place. These children are thus not just dependent and incapable of looking after themselves, but their whole behavior shows that they rely on and are adjusted to being cared for, dressed, fed, and looked after. Their behaviour presupposes the continued presence of someone to look after them, just like the small baby calling hungrily and searching with his mouth for the mother's breast. (1970: 59)

Thus, autistic life involves, according to Bosch, a kind of symbiosis, a bond from which the individual partners cannot freely disassociate themselves without renouncing some or all of their freedom (1970: 60). Even at this developmental extreme, there is a social interdependence that unfortunately involves a form of attachment that assures that a mature self will not developmentally emerge. At the other side of human development, illness-induced frailty need not mean abject dependence and isolation. If the impaired elder is to sustain an identified sense of self, however, it must be cultivated and nurtured under conditions that are not always conducive to its sustenance. The calamity constantly lurking in the shadows of long-term care is that the sense of self in which autonomy actually resides will be forsaken.

It is important to stress that elders should not be regarded as completely or fully formed. Just because one is old, one is not immune to changes or adaptation. The basic processes at work in human development continue throughout life. To be a person means to exist in dynamic tension and interaction with the world and others. Hence, to be a person is never to be fully complete or finished. In that sense, it is a mistake to think that caring for elders can involve only saving or preserving some remnant trace of a past self. Our earlier discussion of the primacy of identification over free choice should not be taken to mean that the elder must be regarded as fully formed. Rather, it means that formed identification provides the framework for autonomous action and choice. The mature self is not a finished product, but a subject who actively experiences the world on the basis of formed identifications. As discussed in Chapter 4, the primacy of formed identifications concerns meaning of the concept of autonomy and what it means to respect autonomy, the context of or with regard to the issue of choice. Here, we are expanding the concept of autonomy to include the social nature of personal existence in the world of everyday life. A model that focuses exclusively on choice is inadequate, because it misunderstands the primacy of identification, whereas a model that focused on identification as an accomplished fact alone would miss the developmental and socially interdependent nature of personhood.

Elders are persons who are still engaged in the dynamic process of change through interaction with the world and others. It may be different, perhaps fundamentally so, from the development that marks the rest of the life span. It is development understood as dynamic adaptation. The ethical task for long-term care, therefore, is not simply to preserve past identifications or some ideal state of functioning, but to find a richer and ethically more adequate way to conceptualize the features of the social world of everyday life of dependent elders across the entire range of human encounters in long-term care. A considerable literature has emerged focusing on this very question, namely, whether past identifications or present choices should be respected, especially in the context of advance directives (Blustein 1999; Buchanan 1988; Kuhse 1999; Newton 1999; Quante 1999).

Of the many features of autonomy that might be explored in connection with the everyday social world, I focus on four themes that provide a framework for thinking about autonomy in long-term care: space, time, communication, and affectivity. Each of these is an essential feature of the world-making activity that is a corollary of autonomous engagement in the world of everyday life. Each theme proposes that autonomy is at bottom an unrelenting effort to adapt to and to shape one's world, to find meaning as the person with disabilities suffers burdens of diminished capacities and experiences the rigidity of limitations caused by illness.

Space

Space is not just a geometric or mathematical construct that is objectively out there in the world. Rather, space is an aspect of human experience. The spatiality of human existence points to the openness and the availability of the person to the world. As Merleau-Ponty showed, the meaning of space is given to a person through that person's body (1962: 98–147). As one acts, one gears into the world, and space takes on different meaning. For example, if one is playing golf, one might experience the course as something to be conquered or to be mastered. One must work both with and against its obstacles and traps. The course is thus a background or field for the golfer's actions and an object of attention and concentration. The same space can also be experienced as a comfortable, relaxing environment away from the stresses of job or family.

Space configures possibilities for movement and action. If one is impaired and wheelchair bound, then access is limited to surfaces conducive to this mode of conveyance. The wheelchair alters one's perspective. We normally (in the Western world) stand to face one another and look one another in the eyes. Yet, for the person in a wheelchair, eye level is at waist level for everyone else. The alteration of spacial orientation results in altered capacities and creates limitations beyond physical access. Since space is not objectively out there, but is a feature of human existence itself, human activities are not just contained in space, they define its meaning. People occupy the space of a room through active interaction with the room and its contents. One can thus be in a room in a variety of ways, such as comfortably sitting in a chair while reading, in which case one's truly experienced space may well be far away in a fictional or fantasy world; or one might be in a room alone and experience the room's emptiness and the absence of others; or one might orient oneself toward the room as a project to be accomplished (walls to be painted, furniture to be rearranged, cleaning to be done). The possibilities are unlimited.

The important implication of these points is that individuals requiring long-term care actively experience the world, but inevitably experience a distortion in the normal spatial relations that define the social world. If one does not leave one's apartment because one is not able, there is a significant diminishment of world. To be sure, this diminishment may be compensated by the use of a telephone or letter writing, and one's daily reading, watching television, and listening to music may augment experience, but not *being able* to go out defines the space in a way that is different from not choosing to leave the apartment. The range of activity normally or typically open to frail elders is restricted. This diminishment is sometimes seen as a diminishment in the range of choice for the impaired elder, but such an interpretation is misleading. The diminishment is itself a particular form of existence foisted on the frail elder, one that requires a compassionate and empathic understanding by caregivers. It is not simply a difference of degree, but of kind. The ethical question involves not the loss of independence or choice as such, but how the loss threatens the self of the elder. Restrictions in mobility not only alter but also create a new kind of spatial experience. Restrictions in mobility invariably bring modifications in the experience of space, modifications that require the individual to adapt and, in adapting or trying to adapt, autonomy manifests itself.

Observational research regularly points to the importance of time and space in structuring nursing home existence (Savishinsky 1991: 188–90). The architecture of nursing homes tends to reflect and serve the convenience of the staff and their work routines. Disease may disable the elder, but the noises, rhythms, and procedures in the nursing home can further enfeeble and baffle her. The sick elder is removed from the familiar surroundings of home, a place where she feels in charge, and relocated to a setting in which strangers assume control. No wonder that elders balk, even more so than others who are sick, at entering total institutions. The stakes are so much higher for them. Sick people normally go to the hospital or nursing home because they have no alternative and they have reasonable hope to come out alive, but for a significant number of elders the move into institutional care is permanent. The institution swallows them up in its impersonal and unfamiliar space. Limited space prevents elders from bringing many of their valued possessions and other tokens of identity. The new location often removes them from their communities, forcing them into a kind of premature burial.

Successively and progressively, impairment, old age, immobility, and death restrict space. The world at large shrinks to a single room and ultimately to a casket. Ordinarily, people live in a number of different environments – home, workplace, streets, parks, gardens, and sidewalks. The bedroom is only part of a total world, often a sanctuary from it. But, for the immobile or the impaired, the world contracts to a single room. Designers of total institutions take on an awesome responsibility. They create for residents not just a fragment but also the whole of their perceivable world. (May 1986: 46)

J.H. van den Berg described how confinement to a bed during illnesses establishes a new world for the patient (1966). After several days, the bed begins to smell. The odors of cloth, bed sheets, covers, pillows, and pajamas become an intimate and prominent part of the limited world of the sick person. The existence of the individual becomes vapid and stale as the patient slips into passivity and dependence. Since others must do things, the individual loses physical contact not only with the surroundings, but also with his own body. Daily hygiene and other activities of daily living are taken over by others and one's usual privacy is lost. As a result, it seems that nothing is left to the person. It is as if one has abdicated whole portions of the self. The experience of enforced inactivity manifests itself in a psychological distancing from the external world and one's own body.

The sick estrange themselves, even from their own bodies. In this way the bed reinforces the disease that has placed them there. In a literal sense sick persons can no longer be sure of themselves, can no longer recognize themselves through their usual posture, their customary and characteristic movements. They can no longer reconnoiter space; they can no longer make conquests; something that would contribute to their sense of wholeness. Space becomes something alien, unconquerable, and no longer to be used. (Bergsma and Thomasma 1982: 131)

As embodied, we define our relationship to the world actively through what Erwin Straus termed *the upright posture* (1966: 137–65). The upright posture is widely recognized as a significant evolutionary development for the human species. In philosophical terms, the upright posture signifies the distinctive orientation of humans to the world. That existence is an existence in essential tension with the world. Spatially, humans exist in a vertical dimension that defies gravity and defines the rest of the world as a horizontal field for action. The idea of movement itself implies a functional relation between vital interests and values, between behavior and circumstances, between position and a sense of place, between action and things in the world (Bergsma and Thomasma 1982: 131) Hence, the sick or impaired individual experiences normal realities differently; they are experienced as cramped and remote or as simply alien. The disabled elder, especially one without significant or meaningful social contacts and interactions, thus naturally focuses on her own bodily processes, creating a very narrow and limited horizon indeed. The attention to bed and body work by caregivers instead of to the person receiving the care insinuates a sense of isolation and reinforces and confirms the elder's sense of being lost or confused.

One consequence of the changes in spatial perception and experience brought on by the illnesses that engender long-term care is that the sense of personal and intimate matters is gradually lost. The sick person abdicates this meaning. Rather than *being* a body, the sick elder finds that she simply *has* a body (Marcel 1965). Others care for the body as they will, but not as the elder wills. Bergsma and Thomasma similarly described the distancing that occurs between the body and the self as the prone body is constrained in an unnatural horizontal position (1982: 130–4). Whether constrained horizontally or in a geri-chair or wheelchair, the impaired elder faces a severely limited environment. This environment is limited not just de facto, because in a sense anyone can at any point in time find himself in a relatively confined space, but limited as an essential condition. For the elder requiring long-term care, confinement is an essential feature of existence.

The normal or typical proportions of reality come to be altered both by the illnesses and disabilities that elders in long-term care suffer and by the social and physical structure of long-term care itself. It is not simply that the setting changes as an elder moves from an upstairs bedroom to a first-floor living room, from home into a bedroom in a child's home or an institutional long-term setting, or from custodial to skilled care within a nursing home; rather, the significance and meaning of the change of place are just as pregnant with possibilities and fraught with peril as scene changes in a murder mystery. These changes are significant because the person's fundamental experience of space is altered in ways that caregivers do not fully understand or appreciate. Perceptual distortions occur as the result of illness. As time goes on, the body itself becomes a part of the truncated environment and becomes an object from which the self is dispossessed. Even in home care, the home becomes less homey and more foreign or strange as it mutates from a place where one lived actively into the place where one receives care.

While space is an essential feature of human experience in the everyday world, it is not a generic element. Space, along with other dimensions of autonomy in the everyday world, has particular meanings. These dimensions are features of the ambient environment that sustain the autonomous life of individual persons. It would be as absurd to speak generally of the spatial needs of an elder in long-term care abstractly as it would be to speak of the needs of a particulars species of fish but fail to consider that the space of the fish is a watery world. Institutional long-term care frequently makes such a mistake. When an elder leaves a nursing home for a brief hospitalization, it is not uncommon to find that the old room has been reassigned during their absence and that they are temporarily or permanently relocated to another area of the institution. Apparently, nursing homes observe their contractual responsibilities by providing an abstract space rather than a particular room or bed, forgetting that not all rooms and beds are meaningfully the same to the elder. This insensitivity strikes one as analogous to the failure to remember the need for water (of a certain temperature, pH, or clarity) for a particular species of fish.

Implications for long-term care

The ethical implications of this discussion of space involve questioning how practices associated with long-term care (1) identify these features and (2) deal with their impact on the elder's sense of autonomy and self-worth. Does long-term care actually impose unreasonable and unwarranted limitations on what is already a truncated existence or is it designed to compensate for or to accommodate altered experience and need? In a sense, it almost seems perverse to worry about independence and choice in a circumstance in which there is very little actual independence or prospect thereof and very little about which to exercise effective or meaningful choice. If I am not free because I am not able even to move about, if barriers exist at every turn, or if I am unable even to turn myself in bed, then it seems that my very being as a human person is fundamentally altered insofar as the basic spatial dimension of existence is radically restricted. The restriction at issue here is neither simply imposed by others nor simply a limitation imposed by one's physical life space, but rather the changes involve the basic *experience* of space (cf. Bachelard 1969) and the possibility of meaningful action for the elder.

The point may prove difficult, because of our traditional failure to grasp the essential connections between motility, sentience, and emotion. As Hans Jonas expressed it:

Locomotion is toward or away from an object, i.e., pursuit or flight. A protracted pursuit... bespeaks not only developed motor and sensory faculties but also distinct powers of emotion. It is safe to assume that the number of intermediate steps over which the purpose can extend itself is a measure of the stage of emotional development... It is motility that makes the difference [between sheer maintaining of metabolism and genuine appetition] visible: it consists in the interposition of *distance* between urge and attainment, i.e., in the possibility of a distant goal. Its apprehension requires distant perception: thus development of sentience is involved. Its attainment requires controlled locomotion: thus development of motility is involved. But to experience the distantly perceived *as* a goal and to keep its goal quality alive, so as to carry the motion over the necessary span of effort and time, desire is required. Fulfillment not yet at hand is the essential condition of desire, and deferred fulfillment is what desire in turn makes possible. Thus desire represents the time-aspect of the same situation of which perception represents the space-aspect. (1966: 101)

Failure to inform the analysis of long-term care with these points is also a natural corollary of an abstract approach to autonomy. The advantage afforded by these points is readily apparent.

The elder with impaired motor and sensory faculties naturally experiences a diminution in her world. Spatially, the world is not only objectively smaller but also subjectively contracted; it is experienced more as a closed space than as an open space that invites activity. It seems hardly surprising that, given the problems that bring patients into institutionalized care, wandering or confusion is such a prominent behavior. Such individuals are acting as if they are lost – lost in a strange world and lost to themselves. This is not to suggest, much less argue, that wandering or confusion cannot have physiological causes, but rather that in human terms the loss of a world that is open for meaningful action constitutes a fundamental assault on the very nature of being a human person. As a result of this assault, individuals feel lost; they do not know their way about. If these individuals are still mobile, they naturally move about, but their movement is without apparent meaning, direction, or purpose. Physiological causation aside, elders experience these changes as fundamental distortions in the very quality of space as they interact with the world. Wandering and confusion, then, might be regarded as phenomena that solicit the concerned involvement of caregivers rather than as phenomena that call for management and control. Wandering might be related to fundamental distortions in the elders' experienced sense of space brought about by their (possibly ineffectual) effort to deal with the motor and sensory impairments that cause them to need long-term care in the first place (Demitrack and Tourigny 1988).

Although the idea of a personal space has been a contentious subject in psychological research (Hayduk 1983; Mishra 1983), it is clear that space has psychological significance for persons. Although the significance can only be analyzed in the particular case, absence of sensitivity to this concern is evident in practices such as allocating rooms and roommates in nursing homes (Miles and Sachs 1990). One's sense of self or personal integrity involves a certain sense of privacy and personal space. We *are*, in a significant and irreducible sense, both our own body and the immediate space we inhabit. The identification at stake here is perhaps the most fundamental, yet it is remarkably inchoate. Nursing home existence unfortunately appears to intensify, rather than ameliorate, the violation of personal privacy and space that elders experience as the consequence of their physical impairments.

The importance of space in social life generally and in nursing home experience is the subject of a significant literature (Altman 1975; Brent 1984; Kane and Caplan 1990; Koncelik 1976; Lawton 1981; Lawton, Liebowitz, and Charon 1970; Moos and Igra 1980; Moos and Lemke 1979, 1980; Ohta and Ohta 1988; Priester 1990; Sommer 1969). Uriel Cohen and Gerald D. Weisman (1990) argued that interest in the therapeutic potential of the physical environment starting with Kleemeier (1959) has grown to the point where it is now possible to place the concept of autonomy in its proper environmental context. They identify three environmental aspects of autonomy – mobility and independence, control and freedom of choice, identity and continuity – that support a set of two-dozen principles for the design of environments for people with dementia (Cohen and Weisman 1991).

One practical implication of these reflections on the therapeutic effect of space on the confused or cognitively impaired elder concerns the widespread problem of wandering. The use of physical restraint is a common response to elders who wander, appear abusive, or are so frail that they are considered likely to fall (Evans and Strumpf 1989). Apparently, many institutions believe that the use of physical restraints is the most effective way to protect elders, even though restraining comprises an egregious restriction on autonomy as negative freedom. Response to wandering behavior is sometimes achieved through 'high-tech' devices such as electronic alarms or, in the extreme, harness systems that tether residents to lines suspended from overhead trolleys (Colvin 1989). Employment of these devices is justified by appeal to the need to protect the safety of wandering and confused elders (Collopy 1995). The conflict between autonomy as independence and free movement on the one hand and protection of the physical well-being of the elder on the other is striking.

Frequently, institutions report that they are motivated to restrain patients by fear of lawsuit. However, the risk of lawsuit against a facility solely for failure to restrain a resident may actually be low (Blakeslee, Goldman, and Papougenis 1990: 80; Collopy 1995). The risk of liability for false imprisonment, assault, or injury or death from restraint is much greater with misuse of physical restraints (Blakeslee, Goldman, and Papougenis 1990: 80). Indeed, studies of two communities that do not use restraints indicate that they have no more injuries from falls than do facilities that employ such devices (Blakeslee, Goldman and Papougenis 1990: 80). To replace physical restraints, however, requires adopting individualized approaches to care. Experience shows that use of restraints actually requires more staff, because immobilization causes chronic constipation, pressure sores, loss of bone mass, muscle atrophy, decreased ability to ambulate, and eventual invalidism (Miller 1975; Warshaw et al. 1982). The use of alarms on the doors to elders' rooms and on exit doors, placement of yellow barrier strips fastened by Velcro, or use of a mat at the threshold of a doorway help deter some confused patients from entering or leaving areas. They do so by providing perceptual cues that afford elders choices to proceed or alter their movement. More staff are not necessarily required to permit elders this kind of freedom of movement, only a commitment that staff from every department are responsible for wandering elders and that caregivers share one-on-one supervision during times when an elder is particularly anxious. The goal is to make the environment as safe as possible by being sensitive to the *purposeful* routine of wandering behavior, not by removing all risk.

The key to a restraint-free approach to the wandering and confused elder involves a conceptual reorientation of caregivers. Staff are required to depart from normal bed and body work and, instead, to examine specific problem situations. Attempting to understand the meaning latent in the seemingly purposeless movement of the cognitively impaired elder allows the staff to work actively toward resolving the particular problem. Before this kind of approach can be adopted widely, a significant change of attitudes and beliefs about wandering is required.

Maintaining mobility and independence involves more than simply assuring safety and security, but consists as well in eliminating environmental barriers that provide opportunities for meaningful wandering. If wandering is not viewed as a problem to be controlled, it can be regarded as an opportunity to engage elders in actions along well-defined, secure, and engaging paths. The wandering behavior of the cognitively impaired elder can be used to support mobility and independence (Cohen and Weisman 1990: 76).

The spatial environment plays an important role in controlling elders or enhancing their choice and range of experience. Electing protection without consideration of the costs to the quality of experience of the cognitively impaired elder is to thwart rather than respect the elder's autonomy. Coons (1987) suggested that rigid schedules and hospital-like design elements are not suitable for long-term care, particularly for residents who are cognitively impaired. The desideratum is an environment that affords a variety of spaces, from private to public. Such choice facilitates elders' control of both their sensory and social stimulation and may reduce their perception of threat to their personal space. Finally, the importance of identification, as discussed earlier, is that it provides a positive and practical ground for enhancing a range of meaningful choices for the confused and cognitively impaired elder. As Cohen and Weisman put it:

To the extent that individuals have the opportunity to make meaningful decisions about their environments, they can maintain ties to their past lives . . . For people with dementia, familiar artifacts, activities, and spaces can provide valuable personal associations and can stimulate opportunities for social interaction and meaningful activity. Rather than being limited to a single 'rummage box,' the total environment may be utilized to trigger reminiscence. (1990: 76)

Time

The second element comprising the world of everyday life that is important for autonomy and long-term care is directly related to space. The temporal aspect of existence is not an objective dimension in which human beings happen to exist. Rather, temporality is an essential feature of being human (Minkowski 1970). It has also been an important concern of gerontologists (Hendricks and Hendricks 1976; Kastenbaum 1963, 1969, 1975, 1977; Moody 1984a, 1984b). Humans are essentially temporal: they come into being and develop as persons in time and constitute their identities historically. From the perspective of autonomy, the temporal aspect of experience is not a frame for choice or decision making, but an existential and social matrix against which the very concept of something as a project is made possible (Schutz 1970: 67–96).

The notion that there is an objective time out there is itself a feature of the everyday world. We act as if time existed objectively. Time provides one important way for us to orient ourselves in the world of action and work. Reckoning time is one way to establish a sense of reality, even in strange or unfamiliar surroundings, because it reestablishes one in that one dimension that assures social continuity, the shared dimension of time. Jaker Gubrium has reported that elders at Murray Manor often commented on or asked each other and staff what day it was. Careful tracking of time occurred more frequently when the elder had a scheduled appointment outside the nursing home, though some kept track of clock time in order to watch favorite television programs (1975: 169). Shared time not only helps define events in the world, but it provides a fundamental orientation as well. In the social world, individuals go about the myriad activities that comprise their day-to-day existence. Whatever modifies that existence (e.g., illness or a special event such as a marriage, holiday, or death of a friend or loved one) has an effect on the experience of time, namely, the typical ebb and flow events are temporally deformed and shaped by the significance of the events. Nursing home life, judging from the ethnographic literature, seems to have no fundamentally shared sense of time, except for the depersonalized institutional regimen. As a result, elders seem adrift. No wonder that confusion is such a commonly reported finding, since the basic temporal structure of reality orientation in the daily life of the nursing home is experientially distorted.

People active in their day-to-day lives often do not have enough time. They are busy with many things, and many interests compete for their attention. Alterations in their schedule either slow down or speed up the sense of passing time and give time a heavy or a light feeling. When I say I don't have time for something, in a sense I deny that thing its importance or value. When I make time for something, I focus my attention on it, and so include that thing within my existence. A child or wife who complains that the father/husband who is working constantly does not have time for her is complaining about the way that she feels devalued by his inattention or preoccupation with other things, even while he might actually spend time in her presence. The child/wife may complain that 'he is not really *here*', in the very time purportedly spent together! Time spent with the preoccupied father or husband goes too quickly or does not provide the connection that is longed for. Preoccupation with work intrudes not only into the details of the relationship, but also into the temporal quality of time spent together.

Similarly, an institutionalized elder might employ various techniques to solicit attention so as to force staff to make time for herself, not simply as a patient needing professional or technical care but as a person needing the attention of other humans (Gubrium 1975: 158–96). It is important to distinguish the tasks performed or services rendered by caregivers from the care that is manifested with a concerned presence. One can adequately provide a service without due regard for the person receiving it. The complaint might be expressed 'She doesn't take the time to do things for me,' even though what is really meant is that the service is provided without affective or emotional engagement. Care necessarily requires engagement and engagement involves people tuning into one another's temporal stream. It involves what Alfred Schutz called *making music together* (Schutz 1971b: 159–78).

Patients commonly complain about caregivers or praise them on the basis of their refusal or willingness to spend time with them. Indeed, one wonders why time spent together is so important to elders, especially in nursing homes. Our sense of reality is confirmed or disconfirmed by others. For people's experience and suffering to be truly their own, it must be shared in time with others. Hence, patients seek or demand attention from staff members or others less out of a need for a service than as an essential human requirement. Being a witness to such experience or, more accurately, giving witness seems to be quite foreign to health care professionals, who go about their daily business officiously performing caregiving tasks according to their work schedule and not the elder's time. The nursing home is a workplace for staff, but the everyday life context for patients. These can be radically divergent (Zerubavel 1979, 1981).

As Alfred Schutz suggestively observed:

It appears that all possible communication presupposes a mutual tuning-in relationship between the communicator and the addressee of the communication. This relationship is established by the reciprocal sharing of the Other's flux of experiences in inner time, by living through a vivid present together, by experiencing this togetherness as a 'we'. Only within this experience does the Other's conduct become meaningful to the partner tuned in on him – that is, the Other's body and its movements can be and are interpreted as a field of expression of events within his inner life . . . Communicating with one another presupposes, therefore, the simultaneous partaking of the partners in various dimensions of outer and inner time – in short in growing older together. This seems to be valid for all kinds of communication. (1971b: 177–8)

If this observation is correct, then the importance of time in establishing a common and shared world and in making possible genuine communication becomes apparent. The failure of caregivers to tune-in to elders deprives them of participation in the process of growing older together, a failure due, perhaps, to health professionals' own psychological defenses against death and dying. The effect, however, is that elders, by being excluded, are treated as if they existed outside shared human time – as if they were dead already. Thus, for the elder to truly belong to a world, she must be allowed to share time with significant others. Allowing this to occur, then, would seem to be a significant way to respect the frail elder as an autonomous agent.

A component of time that has important implications for long-term care is the meaning of scheduled time for the elder. The more important or central a block of time or the activity occurring during that time is to an individual, the more important it is whether the time is self-scheduled and controlled or scheduled and controlled by others (Gubrium 1975: 158–96; Zerubavel 1981). Our basic orientation to the world of everyday life is in terms of normal activities and rituals such as basic tasks of daily living that inevitably have a particular rhythm and schedule. Modifications in such schedules or rhythms create conflicts and problems for elders. Since one basic mark of status and power is the ability to control one's own schedule of activities, modifications required for meeting caregiver needs represent more than a marginal impact on autonomy in long-term care.

One of the deepest philosophical problems associated with autonomy in long-term care is the challenge of constructing a sense of self in the face of disability and death. Autonomy is future oriented. Choice involves alternatives available in the present in order to achieve outcomes in the future. The temporality of human existence makes this circumstance a necessity. It is seldom noted, however, that we can also choose our past. It may seem surprising, but people work at reconstituting who they are or have been in the past by imagining a past that fits present circumstances. The past is not preserved in some objective reality. The past, like the future, is indeterminate for autonomous agents.

Consider history. Does historical research uncover past facts that are there objectively to be discovered or is history a complex process of human interpretation, involving the reconstitution and reconstruction of the story of the past? To be sure, empirical evidence plays an important role, but contemporary attitudes and beliefs influence the selection and interpretation of the relevant facts. This means that the past is an idealization, which is constantly in flux as we reflect historically and as we move as historical creatures into our own future (Collingwood 1959).

What is true for the discipline of history is also true for individuals. One is always in dynamic interaction with one's past as well as with the present and future. The past needs work if it is to be preserved as one's past, at least for the simple reason that without reflection and recollection the past ceases to be distinctively present. Events, persons, interactions, and other things of importance are forgotten, their significance altered unless actively maintained. For many individuals, family members provide the setting in which this work is done. Social rites and rituals surrounding family gatherings, for example, recollect and reconstitute the past for new sons-in-law and daughters-in-law, for new children and grandchildren in the family, as well as for each adult family member. Elders without families or without regular family contact can quickly lose their own sense of past and sense of connection to the present and future. Because we partly live our lives with and through others, the absence of others for frail elders can deprive them of that sense that is tied to shared recollections and identifications.

The family is an important provider of care for the frail or disabled elder (Uhlenberg 1987). This fact points to deep-seated bonds of affection and commitment that need explanation. Temporally, these bonds are constituted not in terms of some future benefit, some rational decision regarding what is appropriate or best given the circumstances, but on the basis of what is right, proper, or appropriate based on who we are. Who we are is based on who we have become in the past. The past thus exerts an important, though not deterministic, influence on all of us. It provides us with a foundation for movement into the uncertainty of the future. The past provides the basis of our present and future responsibilities. On its basis, we can rely on a whole set of skills, recipes for action, or typifications that enable us to function autonomously in the social world. Included with these typifications are emotional bonds and shared beliefs that involve the trust (or mistrust) that individuals have in one another and in their own abilities. The model of autonomy problematically assumes that individuals are isolated. It places the autonomous agent in an atemporal 'now', contemplating the costs and benefits of their actions on an indeterminate future. For choices to appear *as choices*, not in some logical sense, but as *meaningful* for an individual, they must cohere with patterns of expectation developed in the past and must be able to shape the future.

The human mind cannot function if it is overwhelmed by options either whose variety is so great or whose novelty cannot be readily assimilated into the person's frame of reference. A choice is *a choice* whenever it *means* something to a chooser. It means something either in the sense of something desirable, undesirable, or at least something sensible as an alternative. Truly new alternatives are often not experienced by individuals as real alternatives just because the very newness of the choice at hand precludes it from being experienced as meaningful. Hence, we choose and enact a future because we have a past that vitally structures our experience of the world. Without a solid sense of a past, we would be cut off from our own resources, our own skills, and habits of thought. We would be bereft of the ability to function as an agent.

Losing agency is more fundamental than losing the opportunity to choose. To lose agency does not mean that we cannot indicate a preference from among a range of options, but rather that such indication will lack meaning for us. Consider an everyday experience. A person is bored and lonely, sitting in front of a television with a remote control channel changer. It would be descriptively inaccurate to say that *she* flits or surfs from one channel to another; rather, it is the television that presents one option after another in rapid succession. Even though the individual might settle on a particular channel and a particular program, it does not indicate that a meaningful choice was exercised and the program chosen was significant for the individual. Quite the contrary; when alternatives are not experienced as meaningful to individuals' core identifications, boredom comes to the fore. Individuals defend their sense of self from meaningless choices either by complaining that no choice is available in the sense of no real, true, or meaningful choice or by passively acquiescing to whatever comes their way since none of it matters anyway.

This loss of meaning even in the face of objective evidence of choice is an important phenomenon that the traditional model of autonomy is ill-equipped to address. Because the traditional model of autonomy ignores the historical and social nature of human existence, it fails to see that truly autonomous choice must involve meaningful alternatives. We have discussed this already in some detail. The model is primarily concerned that freedom of choice or preference not be impaired or interfered with by others, but is not particularly concerned that the choices available are meaningful.

Individuals in long-term care frequently have relatively little of importance to make choices about. Defenders of the traditional model of autonomy often forget this compelling point. To underscore and stress liberty in a circumstance in which viable alternatives are personally meaningless or unimportant seems either absurd or cruel.

Implications for long-term care

Since humans are temporal beings, they exist in time and must apportion their attention and, in so doing, themselves. One of the basic exercises of autonomy involves the bestowal of one's attention. Caregivers, either busy nursing assistants or reluctant family members, who do not have time for elders do have time for other things and those other things are shown to be more important than the elders. Requests by a dependent elder that go unanswered are valued differently from other activities. A caregiver can do the bed and body work (Gubrium 1975: 123–57) with a degree of perfunctory disengagement that avoids communication with the old person and permits the caregiver to 'save time' for herself. Insofar as activities are routinized or delivered without establishing connection with the elder, they sustain a psychic distance from those ostensible subjects of caregiving. Similarly, the distancing of elders from their surroundings and caregivers in nursing homes can partly be attributed to the imposition of institutional time regulation on their already truncated experience.

Erving Goffman's classic discussion of the total institution focuses on the regulation of normal activities (1960, 1961). One way in which these activities are regulated is through the structuring of time. Of course, time is structured everywhere in the social world, probably less so for individuals who are unemployed and engaged in housework activities than for people in the workplace, but since humans exist in a shared social world, they exist in a structured temporal order. That order makes possible certain typified kinds of activity. It regularizes the routines of the toilet, bathing, dressing, eating, and working.

That order also regularizes relationships, even intimate relationships, with one another. There is a time for work, play, and love. These ordered structures are not fixed and rigid, but they form a pattern in terms of which individuals organize their lives and expectations. Alterations in our standing in the social world cause an alteration in the usual ordered experience of time.

Consider holidays or vacations. One can sleep in. One can lunch early or late. One can engage in leisure reading or sports in what would normally be the middle of the workday. One has time for significant others. Indeed, families who vacation together and limit sightseeing and organized activities can reestablish a sense of intimacy and belonging that often recedes in the workaday world.

In the home setting, caregiving activities can occur spontaneously according to a fluid schedule, but often have to become routinized to accommodate the schedule of the visiting home care provider or the family caregiver's other commitments. They, not the person receiving care, typically establish the pattern. In an institutional setting, temporal organization is more extensive and often more rigid. As individuals withdraw from the work world and limit social activities, they gain a freedom from the burdens of socially determined schedules. In a sense, a person in long-term care gains time. In institutional care, however, organizational needs impose a bureaucratic temporal structure on the basic rhythms of daily life, a structure that is geared toward the workaday world of the staff more than to the needs of residents. When residents are awakened, bathed, and dressed or put to bed is determined more by staffing requirements and the change of shifts than by sensitivity to the preferences of the residents themselves. The bureaucratic nature and temporal organization of most institutional care are not necessarily ethically problematic, but the temporal organization and structure of institutions should not simply be accepted without question. They should be subject to scrutiny regarding their effect on promoting and respecting the autonomy of residents.

If time structures social reality, then the temporal dimension of existence must be seriously considered. If I cannot sleep and have nothing else to do, I am left with ennui. Ennui can be a significant source of patient fatigue. Boredom simply means that one is experiencing emptiness between events in time structured by others and out of one's control (Bergsma and Thomasma 1982: 138–40). Activities that are typically structured in our society include going to work, eating, and meal preparation. In addition, persons structure their lives around special events or personally meaningful activities. For bedfast institutionalized elders or elders with restricted mobility, few personally structured events are possible, especially for elders who suffer from cognitive disorders or confusion. Instead, the institutional schedule and structure take over and the patient is reoriented instead toward waking up, washing, meals, and lights out. Hence, it is no wonder that institutionalized elders attach such significance to these institutional routines. Ask a patient to describe the day and the description will usually focus on when he awoke, when he bathed, when he ate, and whether he slept well or not (Bergsma and Thomasma 1982: 138–9).

Since there is nothing else to occupy their time, since they have usually nothing to do, time weighs on them. Pacing back and forth, waiting for coffee and meals are activities that significantly occupy institutionalized elders. These activities cannot really be regarded as personally meaningful, since they are not actually structured and productive in the normal sense. Paradoxically, elders complain about fatigue that might result from the unintentional nature of much of what they experience each day. When one is engaged in work, one seldom feels tired, or at least does not significantly experience fatigue during the activity. That comes later. Complaints about fatigue are often an escape. Bergsma and Thomasma suggested that fatigue is relatively similar to regression in the sense that both can be seen as attempts to escape, not from the situation as such but from the feeling of being conquered by it (1982: 139). This sense of being conquered and out of control indicates how elders in long-term care are blocked from the paramount reality of the social world and isolated from their own sense of agency and self-worth. Since they have nothing to do or since they are not able or not permitted to do what they see as important, they engage in apparently meaningless motions that can hardly be called activities in the sense of being the intentional production of an agent. Behind the observational facade of purposelessness, there is a good deal of effort and work by elders to cope with the time that is left in their hands, but this effort blocks rather than opens the expression of autonomy.

Observational studies of institutional elders report that even seriously compromised and cognitively impaired elders actively work, indeed, struggle to fill up their time (Diamond 1986; Gubrium 1975). Elders engage in various activities that seem designed to pass time or to fill up time with something meaningful to them. This is not a continuous activity, but is divided up, like the institutional day, into three parts by meals (Gubrium 1975: 161–8). The institutionally imposed temporal structure is, of course, designed around the needs of the staff, not the needs or interests of elders, many of whom complain about the inconvenience of scheduled meal, sleep, or wake-up times. As Eviatar Zerubavel (1979) has pointed out, there are strikingly stable and elaborate temporal patterns and structures in the everyday work world of the hospital. It is not surprising that these patterns and structures have been brought into long-term care with the medical model.

These observations, however, do not imply that agency is simply absent. Autonomy is present, but its modality is significantly altered. Time is crucial both for deciding and choosing courses of action as well as for executing choices. There are important linkages between the temporal dimension of everyday life and phenomena such as reminiscence and reconstructing biography observed in elders (Johnson 1976; Merriam 1980). Reminiscence and telling stories about one's life are not the same as dwelling in the past or refusing to live in the present. They are not evidence of withdrawal, but involve psychological processes related to adapting oneself to new circumstances. Reconstructing a biography and telling stories of one's life are integrative efforts that can provide an overall intelligibility. Identifying who one is, not conceptually or analytically by declaring one's values and beliefs, but narratively through stories about oneself, is a common way of establishing orientation in the everyday world. Stories provide an integrative and orienting action that is widely employed in everyday life. Knowing who one is, that is, knowing how one has become, prepares one for what or who one is to be in the future. To make story telling effective at promoting autonomy, caregivers need to structure their own schedules to allow them to be available. If the work schedule of care providers is so rigid as to prohibit such listening when the elder feels the need to declare her story, even formal time for narrative therapy will not compensate.

Autonomy involves more than momentary choice, it involves choice according to a plan. Having a plan requires a projective ability that entails a temporal atunement. Elders who experience distortions in time orientation naturally appear listless and passive. Passivity sets in whenever agency is compromised. Agency is compromised when the ability to project a course of action into the future is affected by distortion in the underlying sense of time. Elders in whom decisional competence is intact but who lack executional ability because of physical or other incapacity (Collopy 1988: 11–12) also experience time as a gap, a hole in the world needing to be filled, but outside their own power to alter. As a consequence, even elders who are able to make decisions for themselves experience frustrations as their dependence on others creates dissociation between the intention and the object of the action. Even though the action achieved is objectively their own, subjectively they can experience it as alien because the temporal continuity is interrupted. Frailties and weakness elongate the relations between intention and effect. No wonder, then, that elders exhibit hesitancy and reticence as they undertake even mundane actions, because the expected outcomes are temporally displaced from their habituated experience.

Agitated behavior has been defined as 'inappropriate verbal, vocal, or activity that is not explained by needs or confusion, per se' (Cohen-Mansfield and Billig 1986: 712; also, see Cohen-Mansfield 1986). The literature on agitation primarily views these behaviors as problems of control as predicated on judgments about their social inappropriateness, but these commonly observed behaviors in institutionalized elders also seem related to distortions in the usual temporal structure of daily life in these settings. Pointing this out, of course, does not imply a causal relation between the temporal patterns of institutions and these behaviors. Other factors might explain these behaviors. Whether the temporal distortions ultimately arise from physiological processes or institutional regulation, however, is not the question; the real question is whether agitation is a possibly meaningful expression of a disabled autonomy that is related to environmental factors affecting time experience.

The temporal experience of elders in long-term care is profoundly affected by what was earlier termed the *fundamental anxiety*, namely, fear of death. Fear of death cannot be far from the mind of an elder needing long-term care. In everyday life, finitude is forgotten as we projectively engage in mundane actions. Elders needing long-term care, however, frequently are unable to avoid thoughts about the meaning of life and death by immersion in daily activities. For one thing, their everyday experience is radically transformed by their very need for long-term care. Barred from channeling this fundamental anxiety into meaningful daily activities, elders must rely on other psychological defenses and maneuvers as they reconstitute for themselves everyday patterns and purposes. Not recognizing these efforts as expressions of autonomy leads caregivers to minimize the difficulties that elders face in the everyday world of long-term care. Attention to autonomy in long-term care that focuses on maximizing choice or removing constraints seems radically misplaced, since the existential problem of death is entirely bypassed. The very meaning and purpose of care under these circumstances need reexamination. If autonomy is a robust concept that captures actual everyday experience, then it must be made to accommodate the fundamental finite character of human existence. In long-term care, there is simply no excuse for justifying avoidance of this concern.

Communication

Communication is an essential prerequisite for social action. Action in the everyday world is action with others. This does not always mean that others cooperate with us in pursuing our objectives, but that, even in frustrating our efforts, others are communicatively engaged with us in the social world. Accordingly, not only does disability affect one's sense of body and self and deform the experience of time and space, but it affects communicative patterns as well. Communication is often understood as a process through which information is exchanged between a sender and a receiver. In spoken language, both words and senses are exchanged, but there are also nonverbal signals that are conveyed in and through the disposition of the body. For effective communication to occur, it is necessary to have a good receiver and a good sender. What is often forgotten is that our sense of self as autonomous is socially determined in the everyday world in terms of how we are perceived by others or how we perceive that others perceive us (Goffman 1959, 1967).

Communication presumes an openness that has at least three aspects: first, the speaker must be open to modify the message to communicate effectively; second, the hearer must be able to listen (in other words, be receptive); and, third, the message must be understandable, must make sense or at least be provided with a context for further interpretation. Ironically, it seems much easier to comment on behaviors that contribute to communicative failure than to define what contributes to communicative success. For present purposes, it is sufficient to stress that one basic function of communication is to define a domain or sphere of meaning for individuals. A person's identifications, then, are confirmed or disconfirmed in dynamic communicative interaction.

Where communicative patterns are deformed or distorted, conflict sometimes results. When the individual is fully competent, appeal to the liberal view of autonomy is at least understandable, even if not always helpful. In long-term care settings, however, conflict itself is usually not the problem. The problem is a more fundamental distortion, namely, a distortion in the possibility for individuals to retain vestiges of their sense of self and personal worth. Underlying failures to communicate and achieve cooperative understanding, a process that occupies much of our everyday activity in the common social world, is sometimes a failure to express or have confirmed particular beliefs and values that comprise our identity. The presence of irresolvable conflict is frequently a symptom of a situation in which individuals have already experienced a diminution in their sense of self-worth, rather than its cause. Such situations are important for anyone concerned about autonomy in long-term care. Indeed, the diminution of one's sense of self-worth can occur even when there is no clear evidence of conflict, because the selves involved are so weakened as to be unable to engage in disputes or too disoriented to complain.

At its extreme, distortions in communication, like distortions in the individual's experience of space and time, invariably isolate individuals from participation in a shared world. This results in a corollary sense of loss in which the elder feels like a ship without anchor, rudder, or navigation equipment. Being unable to get one's bearings or unable to change course leaves the elder in long-term care in a situation like a ship floating at the mercy of the currents and winds. No wonder, then, that sometimes erratic and seemingly irrational behavior results. Just as a frightened novice sailor lost at sea might vainly attempt to take charge and steer the ship hither and yon, so too the elder manifests similar marks of anxiety and isolation. Confusion, disorientation, or wandering behavior in elders invites a critical analysis of the communication possibilities in the environment. Whenever communication with others is stopped, never initiated, or blocked, and access to the world is obstructed in crucial ways, it is not only experience that is impoverished; more importantly, so is the self (Zaner 1981: 186).

In the normal everyday world there are myriad communicative patterns and styles. Communication with clerks, co-workers, friends, family, and professionals often differs along descriptively definable lines. Indeed, one of the dominant features of the social world is our propensity to segregate or separate aspects of one's self as one goes about conducting one's daily affairs. This fact is important, because the sense of self that is constituted in and through communication is dynamic. Who we are depends on where we are, what we are doing, and with whom we are engaged (Goffman 1959, 1967). Our identifications structure the repertoire of roles that we play. If these actions exhibit the marks of autonomy, then the repertoire of roles we exhibit represents and expresses our formed sense of self. Freedom of action is made possible precisely by the degree to which we have formed character traits and an adequate set of habits and skills to deal with circumstance. Our individual sense of competence thus consists, at least in part, in the fact that we know whom we are and can successfully communicate our intentions in a variety of circumstances.

Implications for long-term care

In long-term care, some of the dominant typifications that support our communicative abilities have already broken down. For example, in long-term care one deals with professionals not in discrete professional settings, but as part of one's everyday private life space. Professional caregivers become intimately involved in all or most facets of one's day-to-day living, including basic activities of everyday life. Even for patients who maintain independent functioning at home or in an institutional setting, caregivers are involved in what are normally private domains, such as food preparation, or have ready access to bedrooms. This intrusion effectively means that long-term care involves degrees and kinds of intimacy with health care professionals, who are largely strangers. This is remarkably unusual in normal daily life. Given the chronic nature of caregiving, this breakdown of intimacy challenges many of the stock concepts associated with medical ethics that are modeled on acute care contexts.

Consider informed consent and respect for privacy. Understood in terms of the disclosure of information before a proposed diagnostic or treatment intervention, informed consent has very little relevance in long-term care (Moody 1988). First, many interactions are neither dramatic nor medical, but rather involve the provision of basic or mundane care, such as daily hygiene, feeding, and housework. Given these activities, it seems absurd to require informed consent conceived as the disclosure of information regarding the intervention, alternatives, and consequences. Indeed, the legal model of informed consent as the disclosure of information simply does not fit the typical situation of long-term care. Where informed consent does seem an appropriate concern, such as in decisions to institutionalize, to increase levels of care, or to institute, withhold, or withdraw treatment, the situations are typically episodic and usually acute. These events punctuate long-term care in much the same way as acute crises punctuate normal life. In long-term care, however, everyday encounters routinely involve matters of less pressing urgency, with consequences that are less dramatic, though for that reason not less ethically important.

Second, in acute care contexts, respect for privacy is recognized as important. The paradigm seems to be that the health professional, who is generally regarded as a stranger, is allowed access to private information or examination of, and performance of procedures on, the patient's body only with patient consent. Intrusion into the zone of privacy of patients is generally seen as ethically and legally problematic unless consent was secured beforehand, though there do seem to be cases in which tacit consent is sufficient. The typical realities of acute care, in which a myriad of health professionals come and go administering medications, drawing blood, performing tests, and so on – often with only some blanket general consent secured by the attending physician and not the health professionals involved directly – are conveniently ignored by the paradigm acute care model of medical ethics. Presumably because such intrusions are simply accepted as unavoidable, they have only marginal interest for and relevance to the dominant concept of autonomy as negative freedom in medical ethics. Since they typically lack the features of high risk and importance that drive the paradigm, these intrusions are presumably too ordinary to require explanation or analysis.

Such mundane, intrusive encounters, however, cannot be so conveniently ignored by an ethics focusing on long-term care. (One might argue that they should not be overlooked in acute care settings either, but that point, important though it is, is tangential to this study. Indeed, one might also reasonably hope that a more adequate ethics of acute care might result from sustained reflections on the problems of long-term care, though that too lies beyond the present work.) In long-term care encounters, the typical situation becomes far more important because, in a sense, the typical is what structurally dominates this model of care. Typical caregiving in long-term care is less dramatic and more intimately intertwined with daily life, to such an extent that it is impossible to overlook questions of respect for privacy in this context.

Patterns of communication thus become important not simply in terms of disclosure of information or the way that information is gathered, and recorded, but in the way communication enhances or thwarts autonomous expression. As discussed in Chapter 3, institutional long-term care adopts the rituals and trappings of acute medical care that encourage caregivers to think of elders not as individual persons, but as cases or diseases. Since the treatment is not temporally limited and since recovery and discharge from the nursing home are unlikely, the elder is subjected to a message that only the most stalwart are able to resist for very long. Truncated communication about elders is not confined to the nursing station, but occurs daily in the halls, dayrooms, and bedrooms of elders so that soon elders begin to view each other and themselves less as unique individuals than as a kind of case, problem, or disease.

One reason why mainstream medical ethics might overlook the dehumanization and loss of autonomy that patients experience in the course of hospitalization is the belief that this treatment is worth accepting in exchange for effective treatment of acute illness. The intuition seems to be that significant losses of actual autonomy in acute care are justified by the temporally limited nature of the enterprise. Under cost constraints, the stress on health care professions increases as they are asked to do more with less. So the ideal of abstract autonomy as rational choice is respected in its stead. Such an intuition, however, can hardly be invoked in long-term care. Long-term care routinely involves situations that significantly affect the elder's sense of self and effectively modify the elder's own self-perception. A good illustration of this point is Robert Kastenbaum's discussion of the powerful effect of statements spoken to or in the presence of geriatric patients. He gives the following examples:

Look at the mess you made! You'd think I didn't have anything else to do but clean up after you!
This one, she can't talk. She doesn't know what you're saying.
She doesn't know any better. You can't tell her anything.
Can you do anything with this one? Boy, what a troublemaker she is!
You should have seen her when she first came here, but look at her now!
The poor thing would be better off going in her sleep.
All of these comments, by the way, were completely understood by the patient even though the staff member often assumed otherwise. (1983: 6)

These statements are not just negative characterizations or descriptions; instead, they function as powerful hexes that profoundly influence the elder's self-experience, which is the core of actual autonomy. The caregivers in Kastenbaum's example were attesting to the patients' inadequacies in a fashion that was not just declaratory, but also prescriptive.

These messages confirm the patients' own doubts and fears. They are instructions to be passive and ineffectual. The reduced dimensions of the elder's world often intensify the net effect of this kind of communication. The old person lives in an impoverished sensory and interpersonal field. Her perceptual experience is frequently monotonous, bereft of even normal stimuli and realistically achievable goals. Coupled with her experiences of pain or other discomforts and the side effects of drugs, she undergoes a profoundly altered state of consciousness. The few words spoken in her presence by important people can, under these circumstances, have inordinate effects. The effects might be compared with hypnotic suggestions in which a person perceived as powerful makes confident judgments and demands on a person who perceives herself to be in the other's power (Kastenbaum 1983: 6).

If these observations are correct, then the contrary might also be true; namely, positive suggestion might be equally effective in the opposite direction. Ideally, every person in the long-term care milieu bears messages for the dependent elder. The question is whether these are messages of confidence and positive expectation or frustration and despair. Ethnographic descriptions of the experience of nurses' aides (Diamond 1986; Vesperi 1983), however, do not instill hope. The cultural, economic, ethnic, and racial tensions in nursing homes are expressions of unresolved problems in the wider society. It would be unrealistic to expect that positive messages and images might be conveyed effectively to elders in long-term care without some significant improvement in either the economic and social status of the primary group of caregivers in nursing homes or in structural changes in society's attitudes toward aging and the aged. Analogously, anger and frustration built up over a lifetime cannot be expected to vanish under the stressful circumstances of caring for an elderly relative at home. Resentment is a powerful and pernicious attitude that infects many human relations in contemporary society (Scheler 1972). As much as one might want, it cannot be eroded by conceptual analysis. However, if positive attitudes are possible, they must be conveyed by actions, gestures, and tone of voice as well as words.

One interesting phenomenon in this regard that requires further attention is so-called *baby talk* to elders in long-term care. Baby talk is a simplified speech register that has special lexical items such as the use of diminutives and terms like *choo-choo* as well as morphemes, words, and constructions that are modified from adult speech. Ethnographic linguistic research suggests that baby talk is not only common but universal. It has been reported to have occurred as early as the first century BC and has been documented in diverse languages (Ferguson 1964, 1977). Baby talk is also truly distinctive in its paralinguistic features, especially its high pitch and its exaggerated intonation contours. Empirical research has adequately demonstrated its presence in interactions between staff members and elders in long-term care.

Some see baby talk as evidence of a paternalistic or condescending attitude on the part of caregivers, whereas others point out baby talk conveys a nurturing message. As yet, there is no clear empirical evidence to decide this question. However, research into the positive or nurturing functions of baby talk is relatively undeveloped when compared with the literature on the negative, condescending, or dependency-inducing interpretation of baby talk (Caporael 1981: 876–84; Caporael, Lukaszewski, and Culbertson 1983). The implications of this work for long-term care are important.

It is natural to think that baby talk is part of the commonly reported infantilization of elders in nursing homes reported by numerous observers. For example, Kayser-Jones wrote:

I propose that infantilization of the elderly occurs because staff who have no professional training and who are professionally unsure of themselves find it advantageous to establish a 'parent–child' relationship with the aged rather than 'adult–adult' relationship. When patients are treated like children, staff does not have to take their life-long accomplishments into consideration, and they can more easily exercise their authority. Commands can be given and must be obeyed without question; patients do not participate in decisions about when to eat, take medications, and go to bed. Their absolute authority gives care-givers control and simplifies their work and routine. (1981: 41)

In a section of her book titled 'Old People as Children,' Shield (1988) reported that residents at the nursing home where she observed were called by diminutive versions of their names or by generic terms like honey, dearie, sweetie, and so on. From the context, it appears that she regarded the use of such terminology to be an example of infantilization. Whether or not the baby talk actually had that function is unclear, but the simple use of this language should not in and of itself decide the matter. Because such behavior is regarded as failing to respect the right of elders to be treated as adults, it is often criticized. Consideration of actual autonomy, however, seems to suggest that this conclusion might be too hasty.

If baby talk provides positive and nurturing messages and it is not employed to manipulate elders, then awareness of this effect would provide useful practical guidance for caregivers who are well motivated and want to manifest positive attitudes toward elders. The demand that autonomy be respected, where autonomy is understood abstractly, could unfortunately dissuade caregivers from linguistically conveying their genuine concern. Baby talk as an example of the whole domain of communicative practice in long-term care illustrates the importance of careful attention to the concrete interactions that make up long-term care.

Some kinds of questions that might be asked with respect to particular long-term care settings include:

- What is the content of communication and language spoken to the dependent elder?
- Does it convey positive images that support and enhance the elder's sense of well-being or does it disregard the identity of the dependent elder and reinforce negative attitudes that thwart actual autonomy?
- Does the environment promote or frustrate communication among elders and their normal peer-groups, between caregivers and the elder, or among professional staff or family caregivers? For example, what effect does the constant presence of the sound of a television in the day room or of frequent intercom announcements, pages for phone calls, and so on have on face-to-face communication in nursing homes?
- What is gained and lost when the elder is moved from her residence into a child's household with comings and goings?

Confronted by insensitive intrusions into their fragile life space, elders are forced to adopt adaptive behavior that not surprisingly manifests itself in confusion, inability to focus in conversation, and a speechless frustration. What nonverbal messages do caregivers give to elders? Staff members who do not sit down with patients, especially patients who are bedridden or confined to wheelchairs or geri-chairs, convey the sense that they are too busy to tarry, too preoccupied to be really involved with patients' needs. They tower over patients, conveying their authority, power, and distance.

None of these questions admits straightforward or easy answers. No algorithm exists to decipher the complex patterns of communicative action ongoing in long-term care. Nonetheless, insofar as communication helps establish one's place in the social world, insofar as communication is essential to establishing or maintaining a world for oneself, then communication must be a central component of any reflection on the effect of long-term care on the autonomy of elders.

Affectivity

Persons develop and change through feeling. Affectivity connects or separates individuals from one another. Affections literally produce changes in who we are, the most important of which help us identify with other people. The bonding of children to their parents in early childhood withstands the test of time, as positive affections help forge intergenerational links. It has been argued that adult children have obligations to or at least responsibilities for their elderly parents (Sommers 1987). Actual commitment to an elder, however, is not only reflective or deliberative, but involves affective bonds. One's commitment to significant others is not extrinsic, but integral to the sense of one's self. This commitment is mostly prereflective, preceding and mostly preempting calculation of the costs of this commitment. Affectivity thus figures centrally in the establishment of the full range of filial responsibility (Christiansen 1983: 137–46).

Commitment to an elderly parent, like a parent's commitment to his or her child, is usually forged in the continuity of time. Typically, one does not so much choose one's commitments, one finds oneself committed. This feeling explains the sense that spouses or children experience when confronted with a beloved elder that needs long-term care. They are stuck without the benefit of choice. Autonomy, nonetheless, is involved insofar as that commitment can be affirmed or rejected. The apparent frequency with which individuals affirm affective commitments to a frail or sick elderly parent shows the strength of the bonds of temporal continuity and filial responsibility. That is undoubtedly why family members provide most long-term care and why nursing homes are filled mostly with elders who either lack family or whose caregiving needs exceed family capacities.

The importance of affectivity for ethics is that it is connected to traditional concepts of character, namely, distinctive dispositions that comprise our sense of self. It is important in this regard to distinguish an *occurrent* sense of autonomy, the sense that is intended when we speak of people acting autonomously in a particular circumstance or situation, and a comprehensive or *dispositional* sense of autonomy that defines the overall course of a person's life. Only this dispositional or comprehensive sense of autonomy allows an individual to enjoy a life that is unified, orderly, and free from self-defeating conflict over fundamental beliefs and values (Young 1986: 8). Such a dispositional sense of autonomy is possible only because the self is affectively related to itself and others. Affectivity provides the glue, as it were, that joins the various episodes and pieces of one life into a coherent whole.

Action manifests the basic spontaneity of human life, the autonomy of persons. This manifestation, however, is not just a matter of gearing into the world, of actually engaging in physical activity in and on the world. Rather, action also involves various kinds of withdrawal from the everyday world of daily living. For example, one can withdraw from the ambient hustle and bustle in reverie or reading. Recollecting past memories, too, is a kind of action. To be sure, these actions have manifestations in the everyday world where they are experienced as moments of rest or islands of repose from the normal course of events. In these states, one might appear passive, but they are hardly states of inactivity.

Daydreaming, wondering, and fantasy of various sorts involve modifications of our basic orientation to the world. These modifications in our orientation to the world provide us with the experiential depth and embellishments that persons cherish. Such activities afford the opportunity to remake the world by forming new meanings and interpretations. Indeed, this ability is tied to the very sense of an individual as an autonomous subject and does not usually impair or conflict with an individual's ability to attend sufficiently to the practicalities of the everyday world. In effect, we manage because we are able to segregate and segment our experience into various finite provinces of meaning (Schutz 1971a: 207–59, 340–7). Movement from one finite province of meaning to another, especially to the finite province that Schutz termed the paramount reality or world of everyday experience, involves effort and the experience of shock in transitioning from the world of imagination or memory, for example, back to the world of daily life and work. Associated with these various provinces of meaning or worlds are specific feelings and moods that make these worlds hospitable or foreboding, comfortable or uncomfortable, familiar or strange (Bachelard 1969). These feelings infuse the everyday world as well by providing motivations for transitioning from one realm of meaning to another.

The death of a spouse, for example, sets a gloom on one's everyday experience as active grieving ensues. Grief involves not only feelings of loss and sadness that permeate experience, but requires retreat, as it were, to memory or imagination wherein the meaning of the loss and the task of reconstituting the taken-for-granted world of life are better undertaken. Similarly, experiences of pain, confusion, distraction, depression, or forgetfulness involve systemic alterations in consciousness that deflect the attention that the everyday world demands. Even normal and routinized activities become burdensome and difficult when illness or disability strikes. When ill, individuals necessarily retreat from the everyday world to other worlds or provinces of meaning. When the illness in question is systemic or chronic or the elder has experienced a broad diminution of powers and abilities, the orientation to the world of everyday life can be seriously threatened. The energies of the self are understandably directed away from routine activities and toward the general task of adapting or constituting new structures of meaning.

Coping strategies, in effect, are attempts to ameliorate the disengagement from the everyday world that illness or other stress foists on persons. To cope is to function in the face of adversity and suffering. The need to cope underscores not only how central the social world of everyday life is to our existence as human persons, but the central role of feelings in the experience as well. One coping strategy seems to involve a positive withdrawal into memory or imagination; other, less adaptive forms involve confusing memory or fantasy with the everyday world in ways that further impede the person's ability to function. Between these extremes is a range of adaptive responses in which feeling plays the main role in constituting the meaningful connections that express the person's identity.

Implications for long-term care

There are clinical and practical implications of these general phenomenological points. Frequently, individuals who are sick for long periods of time complain about fatigue. To feel tired is obviously an accompanying symptom of certain illnesses, but fatigue as an affective quality of the experience of the world is something altogether different. Institutional fatigue, for example, is clearly identifiable: a dull, slow motor activity, shuffling walk, slow arm movements, head bowed low, stooped shoulders, a gaze devoid of usual intensity, a desire to sit almost immediately after standing or to return to bed when one is forced to leave it. The elder exhibiting such behavior is much more weary than the existing conditions seem to warrant. How can this phenomenon be understood?

Fatigue is an affective, subjective experience of living through something. Its behavioral manifestations should not be considered in isolation from the person who manifests them. Patients who complain about fatigue and exhibit fatigue-related behaviors are communicating by these feelings something other than what we normally construe fatigue to mean (Bergsma and Thomasma 1982: 136–7). Failure to seriously consider this interpretation detracts from the meaning of this experience in the life plan of the elder with formed identifications. Actual autonomy is bypassed if complaints of fatigue do not elicit attention to the affective character of fatigue. To bypass the affective nature of fatigue is to bypass the concrete identity of the suffering self, a move that undoubtedly is reinforced by our own reticence to address the emotional morass of our own feelings about incapacity.

These brief observations regarding the affective dimension of human persons and their experiences of the world bear on our understanding of the significance of autonomy in long-term care. Illness and impairment are circumstances that block one's typical pattern of action in the world. In illness, whether acute or chronic, one's bodily enactment fails; hence, one's sense of personal identity is imperiled because our identity is so intimately bound up with our embodiment (Gadow 1991). Engaging in activities of daily living becomes burdensome and wearisome. A healthy person is buoyant and free floating in the course of his or her action in the world; illness, however, weighs one down and frequently manifests itself as a lethargy or lassitude. As a result, the entire shape and texture of the experienced world are altered for the ill person. When illness forces the elder into new living arrangements, the expected effects of illness on the elder's experience are magnified as the taken-for-granted ambient world of life, including the house or apartment, its spatial arrangement and affective tonalities, as well as its symbolic meaning, is altered. These changes force the elder to accommodate a range of reactive feelings and emotions that engulf the self and threaten to completely erode the person's sense of orientation.

Consider the simple case of an elder who develops angina. Previously, she functioned with relative independence and self-confidence. To be sure, her activities had gradually become limited over the years, but the limitations were modest and she adapted with little difficulty. When angina occurs, the whole world is experientially transformed and placed into question in a dramatic fashion. Stairs that she was able previously to negotiate now seem to have changed their proportion. At virtually any moment the searing pain might sound off like some hidden alarm warning of limits that cannot be breached. New concerns become relevant, such as whether to install a lift mechanism, to move the bedroom from the second floor to the first floor, turning a dining room into a bedroom and disrupting her sense of home and propriety.

The angina thus calls into question her typical and taken-for-granted experience of the world and her place therein. It creates problems for her relations with others, such as spouse and children, whose concern may itself threaten her fundamental sense of control and power. It would be a mistake to argue that the issues posed here are issues of independence, though independence is certainly one of the values at stake. The options of relocating her bed to the first floor, hiring nursing or other help, or accepting the help of children are not simply questions for an abstractly autonomous individual trying to maintain independence, but affectively charged existential issues for this particular person that can be meaningfully analyzed only when these features are given their proper prominence.

In circumstances like the one outlined above, it is important for caregivers to be aware that the sometimes extensive and serious modifications of lifestyle that become necessary in the course of long-term care force the elder to try to maintain herself in a new and different fashion. Doing so necessarily involves effort. Such effort is a signal feature of what it means to be an autonomous person or self (Haworth 1986; Zaner 1981: 169). Accompanying this effort, no matter how feeble, maladaptive, or robust it may appear, are corollary affective experiences of anger, frustration, loss, and the myriad emotional states associated with physical illness and suffering. Understanding and dealing with these reactions in a supportive fashion serve both to provide the occasion for reestablishing the connection of the ill elder with the social world and to provide the only way for caregivers to adequately understand the real needs of their charges.

The importance of emotional attachment in long-term care cannot be underestimated. As Timothy Diamond reported, one nursing assistant said in all seriousness 'some shit don't stink.' When asked what she meant, the following reply was given: 'It depends on if you like 'em and they like you, and if you know 'em pretty well; it's hard to clean somebody new, or somebody you don't like. If you like 'em, its like your baby' (1986: 1292). The affective relationship between caregiver and elder is crucial to good care. Without affective engagement, it is difficult to hold an elder as she gasps for breaths fearing that it might be the last, clean someone as you witness her own shame, or laugh with a demented or confused elder to help her maintain some modicum of social contact. Even routine activities, such as feeding or brushing teeth, involve affective and emotional connections between caregiver and elder that are all too often overlooked and undervalued, as the stress on service and tasks impersonalizes care to the point where bureaucratic efficiency replaces any vestige of social or ethical significance for these basic acts of care.

Summary

Phenomenologically, persons are best understood in terms of their integration in the primordial reality of the everyday world of life. This shared world gives form and substance to the individual's actions and also provides a way to understand persons as concrete agents who exhibit complex experiential relations with the world and others. This orientation provides a framework for understanding autonomy that captures some of the central insights of communitarian thought, namely, the interdependent, historical, and social nature of persons, as well as the best features of agency-oriented or action-oriented theories of ethics, by encouraging a concrete assessment of the meaning and function of autonomy. More importantly, this framework heuristically draws attention to the kind of mundane features of long-term care that ethics must accommodate if autonomy is to be a useful concept in this context.

6

Autonomy and long-term care: another look

The forgoing analysis is hardly complete, but our discussion does provide a framework that suggests how a phenomenologically inspired treatment of actual autonomy in long-term care might prove ethically and practically useful. We conclude this book with an application of the framework of actual autonomy to a report of negotiation strategies in a long-term care setting to illustrate how distortions in the social ambience of long-term care can thwart the autonomy of elders. The distortions affect actual autonomy not only by coercion or manipulation of elders, but by modifying the existential conditions supporting autonomy in the everyday world experience. Autonomy fundamentally importantly involves the way individuals live their daily lives; it is found in the nooks and crannies of everyday experience; it is found in the way that individuals interact and not exclusively in the idealized paradigm of choice or decision making that dominates ethical analysis (McCullough and Wilson 1995).

Social reality of Eastside

There are myriad ways that long-term care can thwart autonomy by distorting the experience of elders. One illustration will suffice. David L. Morgan (1982) analyzed negotiation strategies surrounding the decision to move an elder from an apartment to a nursing area in a long-term care institution that included residential apartments and a nursing home. This work aptly illustrates some of the problems associated with failing to appreciate the concrete autonomy of elders. Morgan regarded the move to the nursing area as a key benchmark and discusses the negotiations that surrounded the move as falling into a sequence of five strategies that residents were likely to employ.

1. They attempted to disguise their health problems.
2. They minimized the problems that could not be disguised.
3. They denied that their problem required treatment or that the nursing area was the appropriate setting for treatment.
4. They sought alternatives to a move to the nursing area.
5. They created conflict among the home's staff.

These stages summarize the general path of negotiations. Every resident, of course, does not pass through each stage, and movement back and forth between stages is not uncommon (Morgan 1982: 43).

Morgan primarily discussed how staff members responded to each of these tactics, but initially provided a characterization of the distinctive social setting that staff and residents helped to create. For example, the head nurse regularly denied that anyone in the apartment area was really well and stated that each resident was at least a little confused. She and the other staff members engaged in a continual process of monitoring the residents in order to see who was having trouble. The approach involved suspicion and surveillance. These informal reviews attached medical significance to signals such as mobility limitations, general instability, drooling, occasional mild confusion (e.g., losing track of time), and temporary limitations in routine activities (e.g., not appearing well dressed at meals). This monitoring came to be the main interactional goal of the staff. Not surprisingly, residents were aware of this monitoring of their daily lives and undertook attempts to evade monitoring as their first line of defense against a move to the nursing area. The general picture of the social world of Eastside that emerges in Morgan's description is one involving tension and an adversarial atmosphere in which the residents typically became preoccupied with avoiding being trapped in the sick role.

Although Morgan did not discuss the point, it seems clear that staff both adopted and attempted to enforce the expectations associated with the sick role. As described by Talcott Parsons, this role has four essential features.

1. Recovery from the incapacity is seen as being beyond the power of the person's will.
2. The incapacity is seen as a legitimate basis for exemption from normal role and task responsibilities: in a sense, the individual is not held responsible and is expected to surrender normal role responsibilities.
3. The sick role is legitimated as a special social role because the condition is both undesirable and entails the obligation that the person do everything necessary to get well.
4. Since the natural course of events cannot be relied on to improve the condition, the sick person is responsible for seeking out competent professional help (Parsons 1951: 428–79; 1958).

As discussed in Chapter 3, the sick role concept supports professional over patient autonomy and assumes that the illness in question is acute. The apparent inappropriateness of this model for the residents at Eastside seems to underlie much of the tension that Morgan observed.

The first and most common way that residents disguised health problems was through appearance, that is, by trying to appear competent and capable in public. This disguise was accomplished by displaying good appearance when expected, for example at mealtimes. Indeed, it was not uncommon for residents to prepare for particularly demanding public performances by resting prior to the activity. Such behavior, which might otherwise be described as prudent or practical, was itself noticed by staff and, indeed, other residents as grounds for further monitoring. Rather than supporting adaptation to incapacity, both staff and other residents upheld an apparently unrealistic ideal of functional capacity. Unsuccessful attempts to disguise injury arising from accidents and/or other health-related incidents led to bargaining precisely when the resident was least able to cope. At the point when they were most vulnerable, residents were subjected to the assumption that they could truly engage in effective negotiation and bargaining regarding their care. Rather than a supportive, nurturing style of interaction exhibiting compassion and concern, a business-like discussion of health and safety issues typically ensued.

Morgan reported that the medical staff had warned one woman that her general instability made a disabling fall probable if she continued living in her apartment. Having slipped on a bathroom scale and cut her leg, she attempted to care for herself rather than to admit to the fall. The wound ulcerated and she was eventually unable to leave her bed. At this point, her absence from the dining room was noted and she was immediately moved to the nursing area, where she remained bedridden for 2 months due as much to mental collapse as to the condition of her leg (1982: 43–4). Because the staff actively worked at discovering incapacities on the part of residents, the residents tried to avoid the consequence of such discovery, namely, a forced negotiation regarding a move to the nursing home. The conflict that resulted from the effort of each side to control the unacceptable behavior of the other produced still higher levels of the undesired behavior. Morgan pointed out that most of the so-called negotiations at Eastside tended to heighten rather than to resolve conflict. It is important to understand both why this was so and how incorporating a phenomenologically accurate view of actual autonomy might have helped this situation.

Appeal to autonomy as independence

It is important to note, however, that on a superficial reading, the traditional view of autonomy seems to be recommended by just this case. One might easily argue that the staff at Eastside was guilty of obsessive interference in the lives of the residents, which engendered anxiety, if not paranoia, about the move to the nursing area. In a sense, the staff seemed bent on an intrusive interference in the lives of the residents. It predictably created an adversarial situation in which the interactions between residents and staff were structured by suspicion and distrust. Because of the disproportionate power of staff over residents, appeals to the autonomy of the residents, for example as expressed in terms of the residents' rights to privacy, be left alone, or to decide regarding the style and locus of care, would protect elders in situations in which they were most decisionally vulnerable. That observation is true enough, but it only scratches the surface of the social world of Eastside and hardly helps us think creatively about correcting the problems that arose. The traditional concept of autonomy simply does not address what is most ethically problematic about this situation and it does not suggest ways to remedy the deficiencies. An alternative analysis is required.

A phenomenologically informed analysis

The phenomenological view of the social nature of actual autonomy articulated in Chapter 5 provides an alternative framework for interpreting the situation at Eastside and the conditions that support or thwart resident autonomy. Importantly, this framework does not focus attention on the standard concepts of patient rights and the value of independence, but rather invites critical reflection on the structure of everyday life at Eastside. This analysis will be confined to the characterizations provided in Morgan's own report of Eastside in order to prevent an imaginative, but possibly inaccurate, interpretation that simply reads in concerns that are empirically unfounded. This restriction underscores an important methodological point about the phenomenological framework developed earlier, namely, that it requires attention to the *actual* situation of long-term care under consideration. The practical utility of the phenomenological framework of actual autonomy is to be found in the way it creates possibilities for interventions designed to improve the concrete problems or deficiencies observed. Its primary implication is less to draw generalizable normative conclusions or offer prescriptive advice than to offer an operationalized ethical analysis that is anchored in a close descriptive assessment of the actual situation.

At Eastside, the expectations of elders were in various degrees and manners influenced by the monitoring actions of staff. Apparently, these monitoring activities were justified by appeal to a professional concern for maintaining safety and health – though they could easily have been influenced by other, e.g., financial, considerations – but they produced just the opposite of the intended effect. Instead of bringing health problems to the attention of staff to allow for efficient and expeditious treatment, the surveillance encouraged residents to develop strategies to minimize their health problems. Morgan noted that two main strategies were evident: the routinization of daily activities and the enlistment of social support. Each of these strategies viewed in its own terms constitutes a reasonable coping strategy for individuals experiencing diminished physical capacity. In the interpretive frame of Eastside, however, these actions were taken by staff as *prima facie* evidence of diminished capacity constituting grounds for moving a resident into the nursing area in order to forestall more serious consequences. Although the intentions of staff were beneficent, they precluded or preempted other alternatives that could have preserved the residents' autonomy. Concern was focused on the physical well-being at the price of ignoring their valiant, if sometimes vain, attempts to maintain integrity of self and social functioning. Morgan did not observe any efforts by staff to ameliorate the isolation or negative stereotype of the nursing home for the residents. Indeed, it appeared that the staff shared and supported a negative view of existence in the nursing home.

Morgan reported that residents regarded enlisting support from other residents as a potential resource, even though in reality active peer support for health-related problems was relatively uncommon. Morgan speculated that this was due to resistance against being *dragged down*, namely, the belief that it was wrong to sacrifice one's own health by caring for others, except for caring for one's spouse (1982: 44). As a result, residents seemed to be subjected to unbearable degrees of isolation at the very time that they experienced fundamental threats to their sense of self. Because the social environment did not encourage or apparently permit residents to respond to each other's needs, an important autonomous response to the suffering of others was not present. Staff accused residents who relied on relatives or other residents for support of placing unreasonable burdens on others who were no more competent than they themselves: 'They argued that the health of the potential source of support was in fact no more certain than the health of the intended recipient. They told residents that their use of another person as a source of support was dangerous to them *and* to their friend' (Morgan 1982: 45). This strategy essentially cut off an essential component of actual autonomy, namely, the supportive sustenance that we receive from others in the everyday world. It also served to reinforce the authority of professional caregivers.

In effect, the ability of residents to recognize their own limitations and to autonomously ask for and accept help, an otherwise positive sign of mature judgment, was made into a problem at Eastside. This further eroded the social fabric that supported the elders' sense of self-worth. Whether this contributed to or was an outcome of the social setting is hard to say, but it existed correlative to a group norm that supported the communal desire that the home be filled with outwardly healthy and competent members. It was an ideal clearly exercised at the expense of the declining individuals and the few individuals who were willing to risk the censure of the medical staff and the gossip of their fellow residents to supportively respond to another elder's need. Eastside is a world composed of isolated individuals who promote and manifest counterdependence, the aversion for dependence of all sorts.

Denial is an important psychological defense mechanism that seemed to be at work in the way that negotiation was conducted at Eastside. When the focus shifted toward the implications of a particular resident's problem that could not be effectively disguised or minimized, residents attempted to remove or deny the staff's version of the facts. In disguising and minimizing their problems, residents attempted to reject the need to negotiate regarding transfer to the nursing area. A corollary strategy was to deny the staff's assessment of the problem, in hopes of making the problem disappear. Clearly, the staff possessed superior medical knowledge, but that knowledge was not persuasive with residents who compared themselves with other residents who were more ill. Residents were reported as commonly saying, 'I am not as badly off as so and so,' thereby relying on a lay rather than a professional standard for functional status. Another reported tactic was to dispute the consequences associated with the move. Residents argued, probably correctly, that a move to the nursing area would make them depressed or anxious and therefore worse off. They seemed to believe that life in the nursing area was unbearable. So they denied the benefits of treatment in the nursing home. They directly attacked the rationale behind the attempt to move them, namely, to treat an illness and improve their state of health. Instead, they raised concerns about psychological issues such as depression or agitation that are sufficiently ambiguous that even staff members had to acknowledge the relevance of these concerns (Morgan 1982: 45).

One trump move that staff had available was to shift the burden of proof from their having to justify the decision to move a resident to the nursing area to the resident having to prove competence. Although some residents threatened to leave the home as a countermove, this alternative was seldom exercised. Staff tried to convince residents that no other alternatives existed by offering them temporary, short-term stays in the nursing area in lieu of a permanent relocation. Morgan, however, reported that staff admitted to bargaining in bad faith. The offered solution of temporary nursing home placement hid their intended goal of eventually convincing the elder that no realistic alternatives to the nursing area existed (1982: 46).

Morgan points out that the eruption of conflict or disagreement regarding the move served as a tactic for delaying moves, but it was a last ditch effort. Putting up a fight cost residents the sympathy and support of their peers and led to social isolation, even when they succeeded in temporarily retaining their own apartments. The conflicts took two forms: eliciting support either from outside, such as family and members of Eastside's board of trustees, or from the home's top administrator. Even when this appeal to higher authorities was successful, the residents confirmed their vulnerability. Without outside authority, residents could seldom maintain the goal of remaining in the apartment. The fact that conflict was lurking below the surface points to an important caveat in using the term *negotiation* to describe staff and resident interactions in this setting. Each side viewed its objectives as nonnegotiable, and so there was little or nothing that would bring either side closer to the other's point of view. As a consequence, the process of negotiation was conducted in bad faith from the start. It was a no-win situation, especially for the elders, and contributed to the frustration on both sides. Morgan argued that the basic conflict involved the staff's attempt to prevent the premature death of elders, whereas the elders seemed intent to avoid a lifestyle that amounted to what they regarded as a social death (1982: 48).

Ironically, the possibility of temporary stays in the nursing area was reported to be one of Eastside's special advantages cited by newly arrived residents. If their conditions deteriorated, they could temporarily receive full nursing care within the same facility. In the view of newly arrived residents, the emphasis was on *temporary*. However, these residents quickly learned that once in the nursing area, it became easier for staff to keep them there permanently. For this reason, patients sometimes sought other alternative sites for care, including admission to hospitals when acute care was necessary, even though such alternatives involved additional costs. Morgan raised the relevant question regarding why medical care was not more readily provided outside the nursing area and in the residents' apartments. Alternative locations of care that supported the residents' ideas of personal autonomy and integrity were not seen as potential solutions to the crisis of care at Eastside. A correlative question is to ask what shaped the elders' perception of life in the nursing area that caused them to be willing to forgo needed medical care rather than endure the transfer. Since the alternative at Eastside was a transfer to the nursing area or nothing, a perfect example of the *right to rot* was created (Appelbaum and Gutheil 1979; Gutheil and Appelbaum 1980). The situation was clearly no-win for the elders. The only real alternative for residents as they suffered inevitable deterioration was the nursing area, but the price of admission was a loss of integrity and autonomy.

Morgan observed no efforts being made by staff to understand the elders as unique individuals. The only positive sense of self that he observed in conversation was tied up with the rather abstract concept of independent functioning. Reciprocal or mutual exchanges never seemed to emerge around the need for care. In this sense, community supports of actual autonomy were lacking at Eastside to sustain elders through the emotional strain of the illness or the move into skilled care. Without their independence, the residents were nothing. With it, they were forced to live in affective isolation from one another. The professional care that was a selling point for Eastside apparently displaced the complex informal systems of care and relationships that make up truly functional communities. Since the residents of Eastside lacked a significant history together, they did not build up a shared sense of commitment to each other. Without this sense of solidarity, autonomy is unlikely to be sustained when functional capacities are compromised or lost.

The nursing area apparently represented a loss of the residents' social sense of self. It represented isolation from the active side of Eastside; it represented the loss of the independence that they apparently sought in taking up residence at Eastside in the first place. Morgan claims the nursing area symbolized a situation of dependence in which the resident was under the full authoritarian control of a medical staff that was preoccupied with physical considerations rather than psychosocial and interpersonal concerns. He pointed out that a tradeoff between health-related benefits and social costs is a general feature of transitions along the health care continuum for elders (1982: 47); this tradeoff was highlighted at Eastside. The question is whether such tradeoffs and resultant costs to patient autonomy are inevitable or whether they represent a systemic failure at Eastside to appreciate the tenuous nature of human personhood and personal worth. Independence is hard for even fully functional adults to endure. Its allure in Western societies is undeniable, but it is an ultimately false ideal that can corrode autonomy in relation to others.

A peculiar feature of Eastside as reported by Morgan is the way that the transition between apartment living and existence in the nursing area constituted less a transition than a shock, a shattering shift into a different reality that removed the individual's sense of personal identity and social functioning. The nursing area represented a loss of the paramount reality, because patients therein were perceived to be incapable of functioning as truly autonomous agents. It seems that residents believed that once they were in the nursing area, they would lose the prospect of continuing any meaningful interaction and action. Most troubling is the apparent fact that apartment life did not seem to afford a particularly rich social existence either. Morgan does not actually discuss the quality of daily life for residents of the apartments, focusing on the preoccupation of apartment residents with the surveillance by staff, but one wonders about the richness or diversity of experiences for the apartment residents at Eastside.

Certainly, some residents moved into the nursing area as a result of serious illness and not because of any overprotective concern of staff members. Nevertheless, staff appeared to regard the residents more as patients or as potential patients, even when they lived and functioned in their own apartments. Guided by assumptions that nursing home residents would not be able to make decisions for themselves or function in any way that preserved their sense of autonomous action, the nursing area came to symbolize the very loss of independence and autonomy that residents of Eastside hoped to avoid. It is fair to say that the lack of a real respect for autonomy in long-term care permeated Eastside. Since the staff seemed incapable of providing patients with any sense of hope or meaningful or nurturing interactions, they appeared as authority figures that threatened individual preference and self-determination. Inevitably, conflicts over the move erupted, but these conflicts were the tip of the proverbial iceberg. The real ethical problems at Eastside were far deeper and more significant.

Our discussion of Morgan's description of Eastside involves a reading between the lines of both the report and its analysis. Such reading is precisely what is required if we are to apply the phenomenological understanding of actual autonomy to this report. Simply focusing on obvious instances of autonomous behavior or their frustration, as expressed in terms of patients' rights and decisional conflicts, does not help us to plumb the depth of the challenges associated with respecting and enhancing autonomy at Eastside.

Eastside presents a case in which the social structure of everyday life did not seem conducive to supporting the full range of human potential that is open even for elders suffering disabilities and frailties of old age (Gamroth, Semradek, and Tornquist 1995). Eastside presents a striking instance in which the possibly beneficent concern of staff encouraged resident isolation from those around them. The state achieved at Eastside seems less true independence than loneliness, which can be understood either as social isolation or emotional isolation (Mullins and McNicholas 1986).

Loneliness as social isolation involves the loss of the individual's system of support, decreased participation in social activities, and a reduced sense of social and personal fulfillment (Mullins and McNicholas 1986). Even more importantly, absence of social reinforcements has been shown to induce loneliness, so any institution or system designed to enhance independence could easily create loneliness. Loneliness as emotional isolation involves a discrepancy between the individual's own sense of self-identity, the vision of her ideal self, and the image of herself reflected in how others see her. Features of this type of loneliness involve feelings of anxiety, distress, loss, or sadness. The essential component is the affective experience of being apart from others and apart from familiar support systems and personally meaningful possessions.

This experience of loneliness can lead to or include the realization that social contacts are diminishing, lacking, or are not qualitatively satisfactory (Mullins and McNicholas 1986: 58). Loneliness, however, is not inversely correlated with the amount of social contacts. Living alone, for example, does not necessarily result in an individual feeling lonely. In the case of Eastside, the community setting of the institution seemed to stimulate a sense or fear of loneliness that was fixated on the symbolic event of transfer from the residence to the nursing area. Isolation and loneliness thus appeared to be a byproduct of the everyday patterns of interaction in which unrealistic expectations regarding independence were fostered as a social ideal. Hence, an important ethical question here concerns not only the inability or unwillingness of staff to assess this phenomenon, but their failure to address the effect of the underlying negative perceptions of the nursing area on the residents' sense of identity. Rather than true independence, the social structure of Eastside created isolation and loneliness.

Morgan's description of negotiation strategies at Eastside illustrates two related points: first, the ethical complexity associated with a view of autonomy that is concretely grounded in an understanding of the social nature of persons, and second, how a society that unrealistically prizes independence can lead to isolation, conflict, and adversarial processes. Of course, the true reality of Eastside cannot be assessed from an armchair. The theory of autonomy developed earlier requires a *concrete* understanding of elders in long-term care. Discussion of Eastside is employed only as a convenient, but admittedly limited, illustration.

Bioethics tends to miss the connection between the rites and routines of everyday life and moral action, because it focuses on problems and quandaries, namely, unusual situations of conflict in which we do not know what to do. Emphasis is placed on situations and circumstances in which the individual is thrown outside of routine ways of acting, is confronted with difficult choices, and so is puzzled about what to do. In such kinds of cases, the individual appears to be poised between clear alternatives, uncertain as to which way to proceed. Too little attention is devoted to those great overarching rhythms and patterns that make up everyday life. In these patterns, action proceeds with relatively little questioning or conflict. The typified beliefs of both staff and residents at Eastside led to routines of conflict over the transfer to the nursing area, to be sure, but their persistence saturated the social world of Eastside in ways that Morgan does not fully analyze or discuss. If respect for autonomy were robustly in evidence at Eastside, the taken-for-granted beliefs and values that created and sustained the pattern of conflict would have to undergo radical reexamination. For ethics to helpfully reflect on life as it is actually lived, attention to routine and habitual behaviors and actions must be fostered (May 1986: 56), because these patterns can sustain or thwart true autonomy. Respecting another's choice is but one element of respecting autonomy. One must also attend to the conditions of choice that give meaning to the options that are realistically feasible. Autonomy is thus less a state than a process of being in the world with others whose need for care includes basic existential vulnerabilities. The concept of actual autonomy, therefore, helps us to see that our response should focus on ways of relating with others who no longer possess the independence that we value so highly in the context of politics and law.

Theories of autonomy

The concept of autonomy properly understood requires that individuals be seen in essential interrelationship with others and the world. In this book, this view is developed in terms of a general discussion of the social world of everyday life and the temporal, spatial, communicative, and affective dimensions of personhood. In exploring the meaning and function of autonomy in long-term care, we have argued that autonomy is important both normatively and conceptually. The position defended does not deny the role of other concepts.

The alert reader will have seen, for example, that beneficence is an important value in long-term care that is defended in this book. We did not, however, try to assimilate the concept of beneficence or other values with that of autonomy and did not analyze the nature of the relationship between these values to the extent likely to satisfy every reader. This omission was the result of a decision to keep the theme of autonomy foremost.

Throughout this study, an expansive use of the liberal concept of autonomy as independence and noninterference is criticized on the grounds that it is a legitimate, but limited, political/legal concept that is woefully incomplete for the full purposes of a practical ethics of long-term care. Its most notable deficiency is its failure to accommodate the concrete features of persons and to clarify the nature of ethical responsibilities in the everyday world. In various guises, the liberal view of autonomy profoundly influences thinking about long-term care. For example, social perceptions that autonomy means independence lead to the attitude of counterdependence in which elders feel obligated to avoid anything that appears to involve dependence; society for its part supports this behavior by institutional arrangements that assure that the full price of independence is paid. The liberal view of autonomy is also evident in bioethics' focus on decision-making conflicts and dilemmas.

Elders in long-term care need help with activities of daily living because they have lost functional abilities, not because their choices are suppressed; long-term care represents a response to suffering and need. This response, of course, can be unsupportive of autonomy, but it would be wrong to approach long-term care with the idea that the environment is primarily politically oppressive of elders' rights. Individuals need long-term care because their ability to act autonomously in the world has been compromised by disability or frailty. Hence, they require more and prolonged supportive care from others. The importance of autonomy in democratic societies creates ambivalence toward the dependent old. Their need for care conflicts with the tendency to support the rights of adults to maintain independence. Institutional care, particularly skilled-level nursing care, has thus come to represent a setting in which autonomy is seen to be fundamentally under threat. The development of efforts to secure the rights of institutionalized elders in the name of respect for autonomy helps marginally, at best, to improve their care. At worst, these efforts foment conflict and confusion without ennobling the elders or improving their residual autonomy.

Expressed as negative freedom, autonomy focuses on how individuals want to act and on what they want to do. This focus, however, ignores or fails to take into consideration the wide variability in the capacity of individuals to reflect on and adopt particular attitudes toward their desires and values. It also ignores how their desires and preferences were acquired. The practical outcome of this theoretical approach is that other forms or features of autonomy are overlooked or misinterpreted in long-term care. The outcome is that caregivers are encouraged to look for the ideal of autonomous choice or decision making rather than the actual presence of other features of autonomy. If the content of particular values and beliefs and how these were acquired matter to persons, then an account that incorporates developmental aspects of actual autonomy is sorely needed.

In an effort to capture the core commitments of autonomy, Gerald Dworkin, a leading theorist, has argued that what is needed is a 'fuller appreciation of the higher-order preferences' (1988: 106). This view, and others like it, is certainly on the right track, but it moves on a plane of analysis that is far too formal to provide much guidance for long-term care. The underlying view of the person still relies on an idealization of autonomy, namely, an individual who is capable of clear self-conscious and critical reflection. Attempts like Dworkin's retain an austere view of second-order preferences and the critical and reflective abilities necessary for their estimation. These approaches vastly oversimplify the variegated meaning of autonomy in everyday life that seldom attains the level of this ideal.

The account of autonomy developed in this book has favored an approach that incorporates developmental and relational features of autonomous action. We have stressed the importance of identification. Identification, however, does not require or presuppose a highly developed intellectual reflection. Identification is a complex process that ranges from the theoretical ideal at one end to the opposite extreme of testing and modifying beliefs and values in everyday, largely unreflective, action and experience. The requirement that a self-conscious reflective agent certify all values as one's own is not just an unrealistically lofty ideal; it is an intellectual idealization of a wide variety of complex affective and emotional processes that theoretical accounts have inadequately addressed. The account of autonomy sketched in this book has been characterized as a *framework* rather than a theory, because it, too, has not explored these processes systematically. The framework does make clear that these processes are central for autonomy, both in its everyday functions and in long-term care. Our account also presupposes that affectivity and other nonintellectual ways of relating to the world and other persons will be central features in any phenomenologically complete account of autonomy.

Elders who need long-term care suffer not only because they have physical impairments and incapacities, but also because they experience affective, cognitive, and memory distortions as well. Confusion and wandering are prominent behaviors of institutionalized elders. If the concept of autonomy is to have any ethically significant applicability to this population, then it will need to have enough elasticity to accommodate these unruly clinical details. Standard theoretical treatments of autonomy generally do not adequately address the clinical realities of dependence and long-term care. The concept of autonomy in long-term care must therefore draw on other sources such as mundane and ordinary circumstances of dependence and disability if it is to have any practical relevance.

Theoretical analysis of autonomy has typically traveled on main highways and has shied away from the byways and back roads. This book has concentrated on these back roads, but it has hardly offered an exhaustive exploration. Rather, our excursion has provided a series of snapshots of roadside features of autonomy in long-term care. Our broad characterization of actual autonomy was more like a travel advertisement than a geographical treatise on the makeup of the interior lands. We can only hope that description of the landscape is interesting and important enough to encourage others to undertake fuller explorations of the land of autonomy in long-term care.

Final thoughts

The frailties and incapacities associated with old age challenge families, friends, health care institutions, health care professionals, and contemporary societies to respond with compassion and understanding. These conditions also challenge the basic concepts of bioethics to help address the emotional, medical, and rehabilitative needs of these individuals. Forged in the context of acute care, the standard concepts of patient autonomy and rights admirably illuminate the darker features of physician–patient relationships and the problematic practices in medical institutions. In these settings, appeal to patient autonomy has served as a powerful corrective to traditional medical paternalism. With roots in ethical and political theory, autonomy has provided a firm foundation for the articulation of patient rights. Standard treatments of autonomy unfortunately tend to obscure the deep and perplexing problems associated with chronic disability and dependence. The argument developed in this book has been designed to show that the deficiencies associated with standard accounts of autonomy are mainly due to the way these accounts rely on idealized pictures of what autonomy actually involves. Once these views are reexamined and the limits of their applicability to long-term care are appreciated, other ways of practically respecting actual autonomy can be explored.

Because actual autonomy is found in complex and variegated forms in the everyday world of experience, practical guidance for addressing ethical questions in long-term care should be drawn as much from this rich repository as from the austere theoretical characterizations. Actual autonomy is expressed in a personal life that includes affective connections with others. Not all of these connections, of course, support or enable the individual to fully realize the ideals associated with theories of autonomy. Some biographies and developmental histories corrupt, distort, or disable the enactment of key elements of autonomy. For this reason, the ideal of a person in full maturity of faculties, to use a Millean turn of phrase, needs to be relocated from the plane of abstraction to the complex and fragile reality of everyday life.

Acute events such as stroke, myocardial infarction, or trauma can dramatically and tragically create disability and incapacity that shred the sustaining conditions of autonomous action, choice, or thought. Other, insidious processes such as atherosclerosis, Alzheimer's disease, or chronic obstructive pulmonary disease can just as thoroughly corrode the conditions that make autonomy possible. Besides disease, environmental, nutritional, psychological, or social factors can shape the development or distort the expression of autonomy in myriad ways. Thus, the picture of actual autonomy is more like a complex collage than a schematic or line drawing. It is a picture rich with detail that is experientially established and grounded.

The ideal of full autonomy implies the possession of capacities that form the apex of a broad and tall pyramid. This apex is the subject of the majority of theoretical treatments. Everyday or actual autonomy involves features that are closer to the pyramid's broad base and that merge with other biopsychosocial phenomena. Drawing from ethical and political theory, bioethics has focused on the apex and, so, has tended to oversimplify the complex reality of disability and dependence. Our exploration of actual autonomy has sketched an understanding of autonomy that we hope is more inclusive of its basic elements. Our consideration of the affective, communicative, spatial, temporal dimensions of action in the social world of everyday life suggests that there are broader, and perhaps stronger, ways to respect and rehabilitate autonomy in frail or compromised persons than focusing on decision making. The deep source of this reflection is thus less theoretical accounts of autonomy than the actual manifestations of autonomy in the social world of everyday life. By focusing on how autonomy actually appears under conditions of dependence, caregivers might be empowered to develop strategies for acknowledging and augmenting it in long-term care settings. Regarded in this light, the ethical problems associated with the long-term care of disabled or dependent elders might become more tractable.

Throughout our discussion, we have kept the policy aspects of long-term care in the background. As such, they defined the horizon or boundary conditions for our discussion of many aspects of long-term care. In some chapters they helped define the specific context for analysis, but were never the focus of our concern. Although their influence on the everyday reality of long-term care is profound, actual autonomy is to be found more in the basic interpersonal contexts in which care is delivered than at the level of administration, organization, or payment. Although these background aspects of long-term care are essential for promoting the practical processes of respecting the actual autonomy of dependent persons in long-term care, they cannot guarantee its accomplishment, though they surely limit its likelihood of success. This book was instead written with the hope that caregivers of frail and disabled elders might be helped to reevaluate their practices and inspired to respect the residual autonomy of their patients. The goal of this book was to sketch a framework for respecting autonomy in long-term care and not to elaborate practical guidelines or a full theory of autonomy in long-term care. Our discussion is best regarded as a scaffolding upon which families, friends, and health professionals can construct approaches to the practical problems involved in caring for frail and disabled elders.

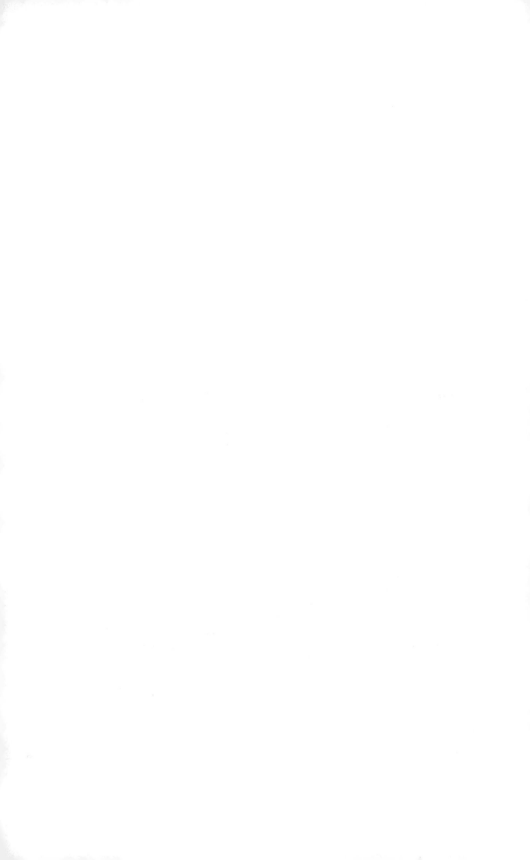

References

Administration on Aging. 2000. *A Profile of Older Americans: 2000*. Washington, DC: US Department of Health and Human Services.

Agich, G.J. 1981. The question of technology in medicine. In S. Skousgaard (ed.), *Phenomenology and Understanding Human Destiny*. Washington, DC: Center for Advanced Research in Phenomenology and University Press of America, 81–92.

Agich, G.J. 1982. The concept of responsibility in medicine. In G.J. Agich (ed.), *Responsibility in Health Care*. Dordrecht, Holland: D. Reidel, 53–73.

Agich, G.J. 1983a. Disease and value: a rejection of the value neutrality thesis. *Theoretical Medicine* 4: 27–41.

Agich, G.J. 1983b. Scope of the therapeutic relationship. In E.E. Shelp (ed.), *The Clinical Encounter*. Dordrecht, Holland: D. Reidel, 233–50.

Agich, G.J. 1986. Economic cost and moral value. In G.J. Agich and C.E. Begley (eds.), *The Price of Health*. Dordrecht, Holland: D. Reidel, 23–42.

Agich, G.J. 1987. Incentives and obligations under prospective payment. *Journal of Medicine and Philosophy* 11: 123–44.

Agich, G.J. 1990a. Medicine as business and profession. *Theoretical Medicine* 11: 311–24.

Agich, G.J. 1990b. Rationing and professional autonomy. *Law, Medicine & Health Care* 18(Spring–Summer): 77–84.

Agich, G.J. 1990c. Reassessing autonomy in long-term care. *Hastings Center Report* 20(6): 12–17.

Agich, G.J. 1991. Access to health care: charity and rights. In T.J. Bole and W.B. Bondeson (eds.), *Rights to Health Care*. Dordrecht, Holland: Kluwer, 185–98.

Agich, G.J. 1994. Autonomy in Alzheimer disease. In E. Giacobini and R.E. Becker (eds.), *Alzheimer Disease: Therapeutic Strategies*. Boston: Birkhäuser, 464–9.

Agich, G.J. 1995a. Actual autonomy and long-term care decision making. In L.B. McCullough and N.L. Wilson (eds.), *Long-Term Care Decisions: Ethical and Conceptual Dimensions*. Baltimore: Johns Hopkins University Press, 113–36.

Agich, G.J. 1995b. Chronic illness and freedom. In S.K. Toombs, D. Barnard, and R.A. Carson (eds.), *Chronic Illness: From Experience to Policy*. Indianapolis: Indiana University Press, 129–53.

Agich, G.J. 1996. Making consent work in Alzheimer disease research. In E. Giacobini, R.E. Becker, and P. Robert (eds.), *Alzheimer Disease: From Molecular Biology to Therapy*. Boston: Birkhauser, 541–54.

Agich, G.J. 1997. Maladie chronique et autonomie: quelques leçons pour comprendre la schizophrénie. *L'Evolution Psychiatrique* 62: 401–9.

Agich, G.J. 1999. Ethical problems in caring for demented patients. S. Govoni and M. Trabucci (eds.), *Dementias: Biological Basis and Clinical Approach to Treatment.* Milan: Springer-Verlag Italia Srl, 299–310.

Agich, G.J. 2001. Implications of paradigms of aging for bioethics. In D.N. Weisstub, D.C. Thomasma, S. Gauthier, and G.F. Tomossy (eds.), *Aging and Mental Health.* Dordrecht, Holland and Boston: Kluwer Academic Publishers, 15–28.

Altman, I. 1975. *The Environment and Social Behavior: Privacy, Personal Space, Territory, Crowding.* Monterey, CA: Brooks/Cole.

Ambrogi, D.M. 1990. Nursing home admissions: problematic process and agreements. *Generations* 14(Supplement): 72–4.

Ambrogi, D.M. and L.E. Gerard. 1986. *Autonomy of Nursing Home Residents: A Study of California Nursing Home Admission Agreements.* San Francisco, CA: Law Center on Long Term Care.

Ambrogi, D.M. and F. Leonard. 1988a. The impact of nursing home admission agreements on resident autonomy. *Gerontologist* 28(Supplement, June): 82–9.

Ambrogi, D.M. and F. Leonard. 1988b. *Nursing Home Admission Agreements: State Studies, National Recommendations.* San Francisco, CA: California Law Center on Long Term Care.

American College of Physicians. 1984a. American College of Physicians Ethics Manual Part I. *Annals of Internal Medicine* 101(1): 129–37.

American College of Physicians. 1984b. American College of Physicians Ethics Manual Part II. *Annals of Internal Medicine* 101(2): 263–74.

Appelbaum, P.S. and T.G. Gutheil. 1979. Rotting with their rights on: constitution theory and reality in drug refusal by psychiatric patients. *Bulletin of the American Journal of Psychiatry in the Law* 7: 308–17.

Azarnoff, R.S. and A.E. Scharach. 1988. Can employees carry the eldercare burden? *Personnel Journal* 67: 60–5.

Bachelard, G. 1969. *The Poetics of Space.* Maria Jolas (tr.). Boston: Beacon Press.

Baum, W. 1980–81. The therapeutic value of oral history. *International Journal, Aging and Human Development* 12(1): 49–53.

Beauchamp, T.L. and J.F. Childress. 1983. *Principles of Biomedical Ethics,* Third Edition. New York and Oxford: Oxford University Press.

Beauvoir, S. de. 1972. *The Coming of Age.* Patrick O'Brien (tr.). New York: Putnam.

Bellah, R.N., R. Madsen, W.N. Sullivan, A. Swindler, and S. Tipton. 1985. *Habits of the Heart: Individualism and Commitment in American Life.* Berkeley, CA: University of California Press.

Benhabib, S. 1987. The generalized and the concrete other: the Kohlberg–Gilligan controversy and moral theory. In E.F. Kittay and D.T. Meyers (eds.), *Women and Moral Theory.* Totowa, NJ: Rowan & Littlefield, 154–77.

Benjamin, M. and J. Curtis. 1981. *Ethics in Nursing.* New York: Oxford University Press.

Benn, S.I. 1976. Freedom, autonomy and the concept of a person. *Proceedings of Aristotelian Society* 76: 109–30.

Bergmann, F. 1977. *On Being Free.* Notre Dame, IN: University of Notre Dame Press.

Bergsma, J. and D. Thomasma. 1982. *Health Care: Its Psychosocial Dimensions.* Pittsburgh, PA: Duquesne University Press.

Berlin, I. 1969. *Four Essays on Liberty.* Oxford: Oxford University Press.

Berman, H.J. 1994. *Interpreting the Aging Self: Personal Journals of LaterLife.* New York: Springer Publishing Company.

Bettelheim, B. 1960. *The Informed Heart: Autonomy in a Mass Society.* New York: Free Press.

Bittner, E. 1973. Objectivity and realism in sociology. In G. Psathas (ed.), *Phenomenological Sociology.* New York: Wiley, 109–25.

Blakeslee, J., B. Goldman, and D. Papougenis. 1990. Untying the elderly: Kendal's restraint-free program at Longwood and Crosslands. *Generations* 14(Supplement): 79–80.

Blustein, J. 1999. Choosing for others as continuing a life story: the problem of personal identity revisited. *Journal of Law, Medicine & Ethics.* 27(1): 20–31.

Bogan, J. and D. Farrell. 1978. Freedom and happiness in Mill's defense of liberty. *Philosophical Quarterly* 28: 325–38.

Bosch, G. 1970. *Infantile Autism: A Clinical and Phenomenological–Anthropological Investigation Taking Language as the Guide.* D. Jordan and I. Jordan (trs.). Berlin/Heidelberg/New York: Springer-Verlag.

Bowlby, J. 1969. *Attachment and Loss*: Volume I, *Attachment.* New York: Basic Books.

Bowlby, J. 1973. *Attachment and Loss*: Volume II, *Separation.* New York: Basic Books.

Bowlby, J. 1980. *Attachment and Loss*: Volume III, *Loss.* New York: Basic Books.

Brent, R.S. 1984. Advocacy designed in the nursing home: cultivating public and private spaces for the newly admitted resident. In S.F. Spicker and S.R. Ingman (eds.), *Vitalizing Long-Term Care: The Teaching Nursing Home and Other Perspectives.* New York: Springer, 159–76.

Brody, E.M. 1985. Parent care as normative family stress. *Gerontologist* 25(1): 19–29.

Brown, R.N. 1985. Contract rights to admission, transfer and discharge. *American Health Care Association Journal* 11(3): 17–19.

Buchanan, A.E. 1983. The limits of proxy decision-making. In R. Sartorius (ed.), *Paternalism.* Minneapolis: University of Minnesota Press, 153–70.

Buchanan, A.E. 1988. Advance directives and the personal identity problem *Philosophy & Public Affairs* 17(4): 277–302.

Buchanan, A.E. 1991. Rights, obligations, and the special importance of health care. In T.J. Bole and W.B. Bondeson (eds.), *Rights to Health Care.* Dordrecht, Holland: Kluwer, 169–84.

Buchanan, A.E. and D.W. Brock. 1989. *Deciding For Others: The Ethics of Surrogate Decision Making.* Cambridge: Cambridge University Press.

Buckingham, C. 1987. *Admission Agreements of Maryland Nursing Homes.* Baltimore, MD: Maryland Department of Health and Mental Hygiene.

Butler, L.W. and P.W. Newacheck. 1981. Health and social factors relevant to longterm care policy. In J. Meltzer, F. Farrow, and H. Richman (eds.), *Policy Options in Long-Term Care.* Chicago: University of Chicago Press, 38–77.

Butler, R. 1963. The life review: an interpretation of reminiscence in the aged. *Psychiatry* 26(February): 65–76.

Butler, R. 1975. *Why Survive? Being Old in America.* New York: Harper and Row.

Butler, R. 1980–81. The life review: an unrecognized bonanza. *International Journal of Aging and Human Development* 12(1): 35–8.

Callahan, D. 1984. Autonomy: a moral good not a moral obsession. *Hastings Center Report* 14(5): 40–2.

Callahan, D. 1985. What do children owe their elderly parents? *Hasting Center Report* 15(2): 32–3.

Callahan, D. 1987. *Setting Limits: Medical Goals in an Aging Society.* New York: Simon and Schuster.

Caplan, A.L. 1984. Is aging a disease? In S.F. Spicker and S.R. Ingman (eds.), *Vitalizing Long-Term Care: The Teaching Nursing Home and Other Perspectives.* New York: Springer, 14–28.

Caplan, A.H., T. Engelhardt, Jr, and J. McCartney (eds.). 1981. *Concepts of Disease: Interdisciplinary Perspectives.* Reading, MA: Addison-Wesley.

Caporael, L.R. 1981. The paralanguage of caregiving: baby talk to the institutionalized aged. *Personality and Social Psychology* 40: 876–84.

Caporael, L.R., M.P. Lukaszewski, and G.H. Culbertson. 1983. Secondary baby talk: judgments by institutionalized elderly and their caregivers. *Journal of Personality and Social Psychology* 44: 746–54.

Childress, J.F. 1990. The place of autonomy in bioethics. *Hastings Center Report* 20(1): 12–17.

Christiansen, A.J. 1983. Autonomy and Dependence in Old Age: An Ethical Analysis. Yale University Doctoral Dissertation. Ann Arbor: University Microfilms.

Christiansen, D. 1978. Dignity in aging – notes on geriatric ethics. *Journal of Humanistic Psychology* 18(2): 41–54.

Christman, J. 1988. Constructing the inner citadel: recent work on the concept of autonomy. *Ethics* 99(October): 109–24.

Christman, J. (ed.). 1989. *The Inner Citadel: Essays on Individual Autonomy.* New York and Oxford: Oxford University Press.

Clark, M. 1971. Cultural values and dependency in later life. In D.O. Cowgill and L.D. Holmes (eds.), *Aging and Modernization.* New York: Appelton-Century-Crofts, 263–74.

Cluff, L.E. 1981. Chronic disease, function and the quality of care. *Journal of Chronic Disease* 34: 299–304.

Cluff, L.E. and R.H. Binstock. 2001. *The Lost Art of Caring: A Challenge to Health Professionals, Families, Communities, and Society.* Baltimore and London: Johns Hopkins University Press.

Code of Federal Regulations. 1987a. Public Health. Title 42, Part 405, Subpart K. Conditions of Participation: Skilled Nursing Facilities. Office of the Federal Register, National Archives and Records Administration. Washington, DC: US Government Printing Office, October 1.

Code of Federal Regulations. 1987b. Public Health. Title 42, Part 405, Subpart S. Certificaction Procedures For Providers and Suppliers of Services. Office of The Federal Register, National Archives and Records Administration. Washington, DC: US Government Printing Office, October 1.

Code of Federal Regulations. 1987c. Public Health. Title 42, Part 442, Subparts D. and E. Skilled Nursing Requirements and Intermediate Care Facility Requirements: All

Facilities. Office of The Federal Register, National Archives and Records Administration. Washington, DC: US Government Printing Office, October 1.

Cohen, E.S. 1988. The elderly mystique: constraints on the autonomy of the elderly with disabilities. *Gerontologist* 28(Supplement, June): 24–31.

Cohen, U. and G.D. Weisman. 1990. Environmental design to maximize autonomy for older adults with cognitive impairments. *Generations* 14(Supplement): 75–8.

Cohen, U. and G.D. Weisman. 1991. *Holding Onto Home: Designing Environments for People With Dementia*. Baltimore, MD: Johns Hopkins University Press.

Cohen-Mansfield, J. and N. Billig. 1986. Agitated behaviors in the elderly I. A conceptual review. *Journal of the American Geriatrics Society* 34: 711–21.

Cohen-Mansfield, J. 1986. Agitated behaviors in the elderly II. Preliminary results in the cognitively deteriorated. *Journal of the American Geriatrics Society* 34: 722–7.

Cole, T.R. 1985. Aging and meaning. *Generations* 10(2): 49–52.

Collingwood, R.G. 1959. The historical imagination. In H. Meyerhoff (ed.), *The Philosophy of History in Our Time*. Garden City, NY: Doubleday.

Collopy, B.J. 1986. The conceptually problematic status of autonomy. Unpublished Study Prepared for The Retirement Research Foundation, Chicago, IL.

Collopy, B.J. 1988. Autonomy and long term care: some crucial distinctions. *Gerontologist* 28(Supplement, June): 10–17.

Collopy, B.J. 1995. Safety and independence: rethinking some basic conepts in long-term care. In L.D. McCullough and N.L. Wilson (eds.), *Long-term Care Decisions: Ethical and Conceptual Dimensions*. Baltimore and London: Johns Hopkins University Press, 137–52.

Colvin, D. 1989. Fall-safe: a falls intervention and mobility aid system for elderly and handicapped rehabilitation populations. *Technological Innovations for an Aging Population: Conference Proceedings*. Menomonie, WI: University of Wisconsin-Stout.

Coons, D. 1987. *Designing a Residential Care Unit for Persons With Dementia*. Washington, DC: Office of Technology Assessment.

Cumming, E. and W.E. Henry. 1961. *Growing Old: The Process of Disengagement*. New York: Basic Books.

Curtin, S. 1972. *Nobody Ever Died of Old Age*. Boston: Little, Brown.

Daniels, N. 1985. *Just Health Care*. Cambridge: Cambridge University Press.

Daniels, N. 1986. Why saying no to patients in the United States is so hard. *New England Journal of Medicine* 314: 1380–3.

Daniels, N. 1988. *Am I My Parent's Keeper?* New York and Oxford: Oxford University Press.

Davis, J.K. 2002. The concept of precedent autonomy. *Bioethics* 16: 114–33.

Dearden, R.F. 1972. Autonomy and education. In R.F. Dearden, P.H. Hirst, and R.S. Peters (eds.), *Education and the Development of Reason*. London: Routledge and Kegan Paul, 448–65.

Demitrack, L.B. and A.W. Tourigny. 1988. *Wandering Behavior and Long-Term Care: An Action Guide*. Alexandria, VA: Foundation of American College of Health Care Administrators.

Diamond, T. 1986. Social policy and everyday life in nursing homes: a critical ethnography. *Social Science and Medicine* 23: 1287–95.

Donchin, A. 2000. Autonomy, interdependence, and assisted suicide: respecting boundaries/crossing lines. *Bioethics* 14(3): 187–204.

Douglas, J.D. 1983. Cooperative paternalism versus conflictual paternalism. In R. Sartorius (ed.), *Paternalism*. Minneapolis: University of Minnesota Press, 171–200.

Dowd, J.J. 1985. Mental illness and the aged stranger. In M. Minkler and C.L. Estes (eds.), *Readings in the Political Economy of Aging*. Farmingdale, NY: Baywood, 94–116.

Dubler, N.N. 1990. Autonomy and accommodation: mediating individual choice in the home setting. *Generations* 15(Supplement): 29–32.

Dworkin, G. 1976. Autonomy and behavior control. *Hastings Center Report* 6(February): 23–8.

Dworkin, G. 1978. Moral autonomy. In H.T. Engelhardt Jr and D. Callahan (eds.), *Morals, Science and Sociality*. Hastings-on-Hudson, NY: Institute of Society, Ethics and the Life Sciences, 156–71.

Dworkin, G. 1981. The concept of autonomy. In R. Haller (ed.), *Science and Ethics*. Amsterdam: Rodopi, 203–13.

Dworkin, G. 1983. Paternalism. In R. Sartorius (ed.), *Paternalism*. Minneapolis: University of Minnesota Press, 19–34.

Dworkin, G. 1988. *The Theory and Practice of Autonomy*. Cambridge: Cambridge University Press.

Dworkin, R. 1977. *Taking Rights Seriously*. Cambridge, MA: Harvard University Press.

Dworkin, R. 1993. *Life's Dominion*. New York: Alfred Knopf.

Engelhardt, H.T. Jr. 1976. Human well-being and medicine: some basic value judgments in the biomedical sciences. In H.T. Engelhardt Jr and D. Callahan (eds.), *Science, Ethics and Medicine*. Hastings-on-Hudson, NY: Institute of Society, Ethics and the Life Sciences, 120–39.

Engelhardt, H.T. Jr. 1979. Is aging a disease? In R.M. Veatch (ed.), *Life Span*. New York: Harper & Row, 184–94.

Engelhardt, H.T. Jr. 1982. Bioethics in pluralist societies. *Perspectives in Biology and Medicine* 26: 64–78.

Engelhardt, H.T. Jr. 1986. *The Foundations of Bioethics*. New York and Oxford: Oxford University Press.

Engelhardt, H.T. Jr. 1991. *Bioethics and Secular Humanism: The Search for a Common Morality*. Philadelphia, PA: Trinity Press International.

Engelhardt, H.T. Jr. 1997. *The Foundations of Bioethics*, Second Edition. New York and Oxford: Oxford University Press.

Estes, C.L. 1979. *The Aging Enterprise: A Critical Examination of Social Policies and Services for the Aged*. San Francisco: Jossey-Bass.

Evans, L.K. and N.E. Strumpf. 1989. Tying down the elderly: a review of the literature on physical restraint. *Journal of the American Geriatrics Society* 37: 65–74.

Faden, R.R. and T.L. Beauchamp. 1986. *A History of Informed Consent*. New York and Oxford: Oxford University Press.

Feinberg, J. 1973. *Social Philosophy*. Englewood Cliffs, NJ: Prentice Hall.

Feinberg, J. 1978. The interest in liberty on the scales. In A.I. Goldman and J. Kim (eds.), *Values and Morals: Essays in Honor of William Frankena, Charles Stevenson, and Richard Brandt*. Dordrecht, Holland: D. Reidel, 21–35.

Feinberg, J. 1980. The ideal of a free man. In *Rights, Justice and the Bounds of Liberty.* Princeton, NJ: Princeton University Press, 3–29.

Ferguson, C.A. 1964. Baby talk in six languages. *American Anthropologist* 66: 103–14.

Ferguson, C.A. 1977. Baby talk as a simplified register. In C.E. Snow and C.A. Ferguson (eds.), *Talking to Children: Language Input and Acquisition.* New York: Cambridge University Press, 209–35.

Ferraro, K.F. 1980. Self-ratings of health among the old and the old-old. *Journal of Health and Social Behavior* 21(December): 377–83.

Fillenbaum, G.G. 1979. Social context and self-assessments of health among elderly. *Journal of Health and Social Behavior* 20(March): 44–51.

Filner, B. and T. F. Williams. 1979. Health promotion for the elderly: reducing functional dependency. In *Healthy People: The Surgeon General's Report on Health Promotion and Disease Prevention: Background Papers.* Washington, DC: US Government Printing Office, 367–86.

Flathman, R.E. 1976. *The Practice of Rights.* New York: Cambridge University Press.

Flathman, R.E. 1980. *The Practice of Political Authority: Authority and the Authoritative.* Chicago: University of Chicago Press.

Foldes, S.S. 1990. Life in an institution: a sociological and anthropological view. In R.A. Kane and A.L. Caplan (eds.), *Everyday Ethics: Resolving Dilemmas in Nursing Home Life.* New York: Springer, 21–36.

Francher, J.S. 1969. American values and the disenfranchisement of the aged. *Eastern Anthropologist* 22(1): 29–36.

Frankfurt, H. 1971. Freedom of the will and the concept of a person. *Journal of Philosophy* 68: 5–20.

Fredman, L. and S.G. Haynes. 1985. An Epidemiologic Profile of the Elderly. In H.T. Phillips and S.A. Gaylord (eds.), *Aging and Public Health.* New York: Springer, 1–41.

Fried, C. 1978. *Right and Wrong.* Cambridge, MA: Harvard University Press.

Friedman, M.A. 1986. Autonomy and the split-level self. *Southern Journal of Philosophy* 24: 19–35.

Friedman, M.A. 1987. Care and context in moral reasoning. In E. Feder Kittay and D.T. Meyers (eds.), *Women and Moral Theory.* Totowa, NJ: Rowan & Littlefield, 190–204.

Friedman, M.A. 1989. Self-rule in social context: autonomy from a feminist perspective. In P. Creighton and J.P. Sterba (eds.), *Freedom, Equality, and Social Change.* Lewiston: The Edwin Mellon Press, 158–69.

Gadow, S. 1980. Medicine, ethics, and the elderly. *Gerontologist* 20: 680–5.

Gadow, S. 1991. Recovering the body in aging. In N.S. Jecker (ed.), *Aging and Ethics: Philosophical Problems in Gerontology.* Clifton, NJ: Humana Press, 113–20.

Gamroth, L.M., J. Semradek, and E.M. Tornquist (eds.). 1995. *Enhancing Autonomy in Long-term Care: Concepts and Strategies.* New York: Springer Publishing Company.

Garfinkel, H. 1962. Common-sense knowledge of social structures: the documentary method of interpretation. In J.M. Scher (ed.), *Theories of the Mind.* New York: Free Press, 687–712.

Gauthier, C.C. 2000. Moral responsibility and respect for autonomy: meeting the communitarian challenge. *Kennedy Institute of Ethics Journal* 10(4): 337–52.

Geertz, C. 1973. *The Interpretation of Cultures.* New York: Basic Books.

Geertz, C. 1984. From the native's point of view: on the nature of anthropological understanding. In R. Schweder and R. Levine (eds.), *Culture Theory: Essays in Mind, Self and Emotion*. Cambridge: Cambridge University Press, 123–36.

Gilbert, P. 2000. Toleration or autonomy? *Journal of Applied Philosophy* 17(3): 299–302.

Gilligan, C. 1982. *In a Different Voice: Psychological Theory and Women's Development*. Cambridge, MA: Harvard University Press.

Gilligan, C. 1987. Moral orientation and moral development. In E. Feder Kittay and D.T. Meyers (eds.), *Women and Moral Theory*. Totowa, NJ: Rowan & Littlefield, 1933.

Gilman, S.L. 1988. *Disease and Representation: Images of Illness From Madness To AIDS*. Ithaca, NY, and London: Cornell University Press.

Glendon, M.A. 1993. *Rights Talk: The Impoverishment of Political Discourse*. New York: Free Press.

Goffman, E. 1959. *The Presentation of Self in Everyday Life*. Garden City, NY: Doubleday, Anchor Books.

Goffman, E. 1960. Characteristics of total institutions. In M.R. Stein, A.J. Vidich, and D.M. White (eds.), *Identity and Anxiety: Survival of the Person in Mass Society*. Glencoe, IL: Free Press, 449–79.

Goffman, E. 1961. *Asylums: Essays on the Social Situation of Mental Patients and Other Inmates*. New York: Doubleday.

Goffman, E. 1963. *Stigma*. Englewood Cliffs, NJ: Prentice-Hall.

Goffman, E. 1967. *Interaction Ritual: Essays on Face-to-Face Behavior*. Garden City, NY: Anchor Books.

Graebner, W. 1980. *A History of Retirement*. New Haven, CT: Yale University Press.

Grimshaw, J. 1988. Autonomy and identity in feminist thinking. In M. Griffiths and M. Whitford (eds.), *Feminist Perspectives in Philosophy*. Bloomington, IN: Indiana University Press, 98–108.

Gruman, G. 1978. Cultural origins of present-day 'age-ism': the modernization of the life cycle. In S.F. Spicker, K.M. Woodward, and D.D. Van Tassel (eds.), *Aging and the Elderly: Humanistic Perspectives in Gerontology*. Atlantic Highlands, NJ: Humanities Press, 359–87.

Gubrium, J.F. 1975. *Living and Dying at Murray Manor*. New York: St Martin's Press.

Gubrium, J.F. 1982. Fictive family: everyday usage, analytic, and human service considerations. *American Anthropologist* 84: 878–85.

Gubrium, J.F. and D.R. Buckholdt. 1977. *Toward Maturity*. San Francisco, CA: Jossey-Bass.

Gutheil, T.G. and P.S. Appelbaum. 1980. The patient always pays: reflections on the Boston State case and the right to rot. *Man and Medicine* 5: 3–11.

Guttman, D. 1976. Alternatives to disengagement among the old men of the Highland Druze. In J.F. Gubrium (ed.), *Time, Roles and Self in Old Age*. New York: Human Sciences Press, 88–108.

Halper, T. 1978. Paternalism and the elderly. In S.F. Spicker, K.M. Woodward, and D.D. Van Tassel (eds.), *Aging and the Elderly: Humanistic Perspectives in Gerontology*. Atlantic Highlands, NJ: Humanities Press, 321–39.

Hare, R.M. 1972. *The Language of Morals*. Oxford: Oxford University Press.

Harlow, H.F. and M.K. Harlow. 1962. Social deprivation in monkeys. *Scientific American* 207(5): 137–46.

Harrell, S. 1979. Growing old in rural Taiwan. In P.T. Amoss and S. Harrell (eds.), *Other Ways of Growing Old: Anthropological Perspectives.* Stanford, CA: Stanford University Press, 193–210.

Hauerwas, S.J. 1981. *A Community of Character.* Notre Dame, IN: University of Notre Dame Press.

Hauerwas, S.J. 1982. Authority and the profession of medicine. In G.J. Agich (ed.), *Responsibility in Health Care.* Dordrecht, Holland: D. Reidel, 83–104.

Havighurst, R. 1956. *Psychological Aspects of Aging.* Washington, DC: American Psychological Association.

Haworth, L. 1986. *Autonomy: An Essay in Philosophical Psychology and Ethics.* New Haven, CT: Yale University Press.

Hayduk, L.A. 1983. Personal space: where we now stand. *Psychological Bulletin* 94(2): 293–335.

Hegeman, C. and S. Tobin. 1988. Enhancing the autonomy of mentally impaired nursing home residents. *Gerontologist* 28(Supplement, June): 71–5.

Heidegger, M. 1962. *Being and Time.* J. Macquarrie and E. Robinson (trs.). New York and Evanston: Harper & Row.

Held, V. 1987. Feminism and moral theory. In E. Feder Kittay and D.T. Meyers (eds.), *Women and Moral Theory.* Totowa, NJ: Rowan & Littlefield, 111–28.

Hendricks, C.D. and J. Hendricks. 1976. Concepts of time and temporal construction among the aged, with implications for research. In J.F. Gubrium (ed.), *Time, Roles and Self in Old Age.* New York: Human Sciences Press, 13–49.

Henry, J. 1963. *Culture Against Man.* New York: Vintage Books.

Hing, E. 1987. Use of nursing homes by the elderly: preliminary data from 1985 National Nursing Home Survey. Advance Data From Vital and Health Statistics, No. 135. Hyattsville, MD: National Center For Health Statistics, Public Health Service.

Hofland, B.F. 1988. Autonomy and long term care: background issues and a programmatic response. *Gerontologist* 28(Supplement June): 3–9.

Hofland, B.F. 1990. Introduction. *Generations* 14(Supplement): 5–8.

Holmberg, A. 1969. *Nomads of the Long Bow: Siriono of Eastern Bolivia.* Garden City, NY: Doubleday.

Holmes, L. and E. Rhoads. 1983. Aging and change in Samoa. In J. Sokolovsky (ed.), *Growing Old in Different Societies: Cross-Cultural Perspectives.* Belmont, CA: Wadsworth, 119–29.

Jameton, A. 1988. In the borderlands of autonomy: responsibility in long-term care facilities. *Gerontologist* 28(Supplement, June): 18–23.

Jameton, A. 1990. Let my persons go! Restraints of the trade: case commentary. In R.A. Kane and A.L. Caplan (eds.), *Everyday Ethics: Resolving Dilemmas in Nursing Home Life.* New York: Springer, 167–77.

Jeffrey, R. 1974. Preference among preferences. *Journal of Philosophy* 71(13): 377–91.

Johnson, M. 1976. That was your life: a biographical approach to later life. In J.N.A. Munnichs and W. van den Heuvel (eds.), *Dependency or Interdependency in Old Age.* The Hague: Martinus Nijhoff, 147–61.

Johnson, M. 1987. *The Body in the Mind and the Bodily Basis of Meaning, Imagination, and Reason.* Chicago: University of Chicago Press.

Jonas, H. 1966. *The Phenomenon of Life: Toward a Philosophical Biology.* New York: Dell.

Judicial Council of the American Medical Association. 1984. *Current Opinions of the Judicial Council of the American Medical Association – 1984.* Chicago, IL: American Medical Association.

Kaminsky, M. 1984. *The Uses of Reminiscence.* New York: Haworth Press.

Kane, R.A. 1990. Everyday life in nursing homes: 'the way things are'. In R.A. Kane and A.L. Caplan (eds.), *Everyday Ethics: Resolving Dilemmas in Nursing Home Life.* New York: Springer, 3–20.

Kane, R.A. 1995. Decision making, care plans, and life plans in long-term care: can case managers take account of clients' values and preferences? In L.D. McCullough and N.L. Wilson (eds.), *Long-term Care Decisions: Ethical and Conceptual Dimensions.* Baltimore and London: Johns Hopkins University Press, 87–109.

Kane, R.A. and A.L. Caplan (eds.). 1990. *Everyday Ethics: Resolving Dilemmas in Nursing Home Life.* New York: Springer.

Kane, R.A., I.C. Freeman, A.L. Caplan, M.A. Aroskar, and E.K. Urv-Wong. 1990. Everyday autonomy in nursing homes. *Generations* 14(Supplement): 69–71.

Kane, R.L. and R.A. Kane. 1978. Care of the aged: old problems in need of new solutions. *Science* 200(4344): 913–19.

Kane, R.L. and R.A. Kane. 1990. The impact of long-term-care financing on personal autonomy. *Generations* 14(Supplement): 86–9.

Kapp, M.B. 1985. Ethics vs. fear of malpractice. *Generations* 10(2): 18–20.

Kapp, M.B. 1987. *Preventing Malpractice in Long Term Care: Strategies for Risk Management.* New York: Springer.

Kapp, M.B. 1990. Home care client-centered systems: consumer choice vs. protection. *Generations* 14(Supplement): 33–6.

Kastenbaum, R. 1963. Cognitive and personal futurity in later life. *Journal of Individual Psychology* 19: 216–22.

Kastenbaum, R. 1969. The foreshortened life perspective. *Geriatrics* 24: 126–33.

Kastenbaum, R. 1975. Time, death and ritual in old age. In J.D. Fraser and N. Lawrence (eds.), *The Study of Time II: Proceedings of the Second Conference of the International Society for the Study of Time, Lake Yamanaka – Japan.* New York: Springer-Verlag, 20–38.

Kastenbaum, R. 1977. Memories of tomorrow: on the interpenetrations of time in later life. In B.S. Gorman and E.E. Westman (eds.), *The Personal Experience of Time.* New York and London: Plenum Press, 193–215.

Kastenbaum, R. 1983. Can the clinical milieu be therapeutic? In G.D. Rowles and R.J. Ohta (eds.), *Aging and Milieu: Environmental Perspectives on Growing Old.* New York: Academic Press, 3–15.

Katz, S., L.G. Branch, M.H. Branson, J.A. Papsidero, J.C. Beck, and D.S. Greer. 1983. Active life expectancy. *New England Journal of Medicine* 309(20): 1218–24.

Kayser-Jones, J.S. 1981. *Old, Alone and Neglected: Care of the Aged in the United States and Scotland.* Berkeley, CA: University of California Press.

Keeler, E.B., R.L. Kane, and D.H. Solomon. 1981. Short- and long-term residents of nursing homes. *Medical Care* 19: 363–9.

Kegley, J.A.K. 1999. Community, autonomy, and managed care. In G. McGee (ed.), *Pragmatic Bioethics*. Nashville, TN: Vanderbilt University Press, 204–27.

Kelly, M.P. and D. May. 1982. Good and bad patients: a review of the literature and a theoretical critique. *Journal of Advanced Nursing* 7: 147–56.

Kemper, P. and C. Murtaugh. 1991. Life time use of nursing home care. *New England Journal of Medicine* 324(9): 595–600.

Kidd, D. 1904. *The Sensual Kaffir*. London: A. & C. Black.

Kiefer, C.W. 1988. *The Mantle of Maturity: A History of Ideas About Character Development*. Albany, NY: State University of New York Press.

Kinsella, K. and V.A. Velkoff. 2001. *U.S. Census Bureau, Series P95/01–1, An Aging World: 2001*. Washington, DC: US Government Printing Office.

Kittay, E.F. 1999. *Love's Labor: Essays on Women, Equality, and Dependence*. New York: Routledge.

Kittay, E.F. and D.T. Meyers (eds.). 1987. *Woman and Moral Theory*. Totowa, NJ: Rowan & Littlefield.

Kleemeier, R.W. 1959. Behavior and the organization of the bodily and the external environment. In J.E. Birren (ed.), *Handbook of Aging and the Individual*. Chicago: University of Chicago Press, 400–51.

Koch, S. 1971. The image of man in encounter group therapy. *Journal of Humanistic Psychology* II: 109–28.

Kohlberg, L. 1971. Stages of moral development as a basis for moral education. In E.V. Sullivan (ed.), *Moral Education*. Toronto: University of Toronto Press, 23–92.

Koncelik, J. 1976. *Designing the Open Nursing Home*. Stroudsburg, PA: Dowden, Hutchingson and Ross.

Kovar, M.G. 1977. Health of the elderly and the use of health services. *Public Health Report* 92: 9–19.

Kuhse, H. 1999. Some reflections on the problem of advance directives, personhood, and personal identity. *Kennedy Institute of Ethics Journal*. 9(4): 347–64.

Ladd, J. 1978. Legalism and medical ethics. In J.W. Davis, B. Hoffmaster, and S. Shorten (eds.), *Contemporary Issues in Biomedical Ethics*. Clifton, NJ: Humana Press, 1–35.

Laird, C. 1979. *Limbo: A Memoir of Life in a Nursing Home by a Survivor*. Novato, CA: Chandler and Sharp.

Larmore, C.E. 1987. *Patterns of Moral Complexity*. Cambridge: Cambridge University Press.

Larsen, E.B., B. Lo, and N.E. Williams. 1986. Evaluation and care of elderly patients with dementia. *Journal of General Internal Medicine* 1: 116–26.

Lawton, A.P. 1981. *Environment and Aging*. Monterey, CA: Brooks-Cole.

Lawton, M.P., B. Liebowitz, and H. Charon. 1970. Physical structure and the behavior of senile patients following ward remodeling. *Aging and Human Development* 1: 231–9.

Legal Services for the Elderly. 1983. *Illegal and Questionable Terms in Nursing Home Resident Contracts: A Report to the Nursing Home Ombudsman*. Augusta, ME: Maine Committee on Aging.

Leidel, R. 1995. Effects of population aging on health care expenditure and financing: some illustrations. In D. Callahan, R.H.J. ter Meulen, and E. Topinkova (eds.),

A World Growing Old: The Coming Health Care Challenges. Washington, DC: Georgetown University Press, 49–61.

Lerner, G. 1986. *The Creation of Patriarchy.* New York: Oxford University Press.

Levinsky, N.G. 1984. The doctor's master. *New England Journal of Medicine* 311(24): 1573–5.

Lidz, C.W., P.S. Appelbaum, and A. Meisel. 1988. Two models of implementing the idea of informed consent. *Archives of Internal Medicine* 148: 1385–9.

Lidz, C.W., L. Fischer, and R.M. Arnold. 1990. *An Ethnographic Study of the Erosion of Autonomy in Long-Term Care.* A Final Report to the Retirement Research Foundation, Chicago, IL.

Lidz, C.W., L. Fischer, and R.M. Arnold. 1992. *The Erosion of Autonomy in Long-Term Care.* New York: Oxford University Press.

Lindeman, C.A. and B. van Aernham. 1971. Nursing intervention with the presurgical patients. *Nursing Research* 20(4): 319–32.

Locke, J. 1980. *Second Treatise of Government.* C.B. Macpherson (ed.). Indianapolis, IN: Hackett.

MacCallum, G. 1967. Negative and positive freedom. *Philosophical Review* 76: 312–34.

Mackenzie, C. and N. Stoljar (eds.). 2000. *Relational Autonomy: Feminist Perspectives on Autonomy, Agency and the Social Self.* New York: Columbia University Press.

MacIntyre, A. 1977. Patients as agents. In S.F. Spicker and H.T. Engelhardt Jr (eds.), *Philosophical Medical Ethics: Its Nature and Significance.* Dordrecht, Holland: D. Reidel, 197–212.

MacIntyre, A. 1981. *After Virtue: A Study in Moral Theory.* Notre Dame, IN: University of Notre Dame Press.

MacIntyre, A. 1988. *Whose Justice? Which Rationality?* Notre Dame, IN: University of Notre Dame Press.

Macklin, R. 1983a. Problems of informed consent with the cognitively impaired. In D.W. Pfaff (ed.), *Brain and Behavior.* New York: Springer-Verlag, 23–40.

Macklin, R. 1983b. Treatment refusals: autonomy, paternalism and the 'best interest' of the patient. In D.W. Pfaff (ed.), *Brain and Behavior.* New York: Springer-Verlag, 41–56.

Macklin, R. 1990. Good citizen, bad citizen: case commentary. In R.A. Kane and A.L. Caplan (eds.), *Everyday Ethics: Resolving Dilemmas in Nursing Home Life.* New York: Springer, 60–70.

Mahowald, M.B. 1987. Sex-role stereotypes in medicine. *Hypatia* 2(2): 21–38.

Marcel, G. 1965. *Being and Having.* K. Farrer (tr.). New York: Harper Row.

May, W.F. 1975. Code, covenant, contract, or philanthropy. *Hastings Center Report* 5(December): 29–38.

May, W.F. 1982. Who cares for the elderly? *Hastings Center Report* 12(6): 31–7.

May, W.F. 1986. The virtues and vices of the elderly. In T.R. Cole and S. Gadow (eds.), *What Does it Mean to Grow Old? Reflections from the Humanities.* Durham, NC: Duke University Press, 43–61.

McCullough, L.B. and S. Wear. 1985. Respect for autonomy and medical paternalism reconsidered. *Theoretical Medicine* 6: 295–308.

McCullough, L.D. and N.L. Wilson (eds.). 1995. *Long-term Care Decisions: Ethical and Conceptual Dimensions.* Baltimore and London: Johns Hopkins University Press.

Mendelson, M. 1975. *Tender Loving Greed.* New York: Vintage.

Merleau-Ponty, M. 1962. *The Phenomenology of Perception.* C. Smith (tr.). London: Routledge & Kegan Paul.

Merleau-Ponty, M. 1967. *The Structure of Behavior.* A.L. Fisher (tr.). Boston, MA: Beacon Press.

Merriam, S. 1980. The concept and function of reminiscence: a review of research. *Gerontologist* 20(5): 604–8.

Meyers, D.T. 1987. The socialized individual and individual autonomy: an intersection between philosophy and psychology. In E.F. Kittay and D.T. Meyers (eds.), *Women and Moral Theory.* Totowa, NJ: Rowan & Littlefield, 139–53.

Miles, S.H. 1988. Paternalism, family duties, and my Aunt Maude. *Journal of the American Medical Association* 259(May 6): 2582–3.

Miles, S.H. and G.A. Sachs. 1990. Roommates in nursing homes case commentary: accommodating room and roommate preferences. In A.K. Rosalie and A.L. Caplan (eds.), *Everyday Ethics: Resolving Dilemmas in Nursing Home Life.* New York: Springer, 92–9.

Mill, J.S. 1978. *On Liberty.* Indianapolis, IN: Hackett.

Miller, M. 1975. Iatrogenic and nurisgenic effects of prolonged immobilization of the ill aged. *Journal of the American Geriatrics Society* 23(8): 360–9.

Minkowski, E. 1970. *Lived Time: Phenomenological and Psychopathological Studies.* N. Metzel (tr.). Evanston, IL: Northwestern University Press.

Mishra, P.K. 1983. Proxemics: theory and research. *Perspectives in Psychological Researches* 6: 10–15.

Moody, H.R. 1984a. A bibliography on reminiscence and life review. In M. Kaminsky (ed.), *The Uses of Reminiscence: New Ways of Working With Older Adults.* New York: Haworth Press, 231–6.

Moody, H.R. 1984b. Reminiscence and the recovery of the public world. In M. Kaminsky (ed.), *The Uses of Reminiscence: New Ways of Working With Older Adults.* New York: Haworth Press, 157–66.

Moody, H.R. 1988. From informed consent to negotiated consent. *Gerontologist* 28(Supplement, June): 64–70.

Moos, R.H. and A. Igra. 1980. Determinants of the social environments of sheltered care environments. *Journal of Health and Social Behavior* 21(1): 88–98.

Moos, R.H. and S. Lemke. 1979. *Multiphasic Environmental Assessment Procedure (MEAP): Preliminary Manual.* Social Ecology Laboratory, Palo Alto, CA: Stanford University and the Veterans Administration Medical Center.

Moos, R.H. and S. Lemke. 1980. Assessing the physical and architectural features of sheltered care settings. *Journal of Gerontology* 35(4): 571–83.

Morford, T.G. 1988. Nursing home regulation: history and expectations. *Health Care Financing Review* (Annual Supplement): 129–32.

Morgan, D.L. 1982. Failing health and the desire for independence: two conflicting aspects of health care in old age. *Social Problems* 30(October): 40–50.

Mullins, L.C. and N. McNicholas. 1986. Loneliness among the elderly: issues and considerations for professionals in aging. *Gerontology and Geriatrics Education* 7(Fall): 55–65.

Nagel, T. 1986. *The View from Nowhere.* Oxford: Oxford University Press.

Neeley, W. 1974. Freedom and desire. *Philosophical Review* 83: 32–54.

Nemore, P. 1985. Illegal terms in nursing home admissions contracts. *Clearinghouse Review* 18: 1165–9.

Neu, J. 1975. Thought, theory, and therapy. *Psychoanalysis & Contemporary Science* 4: 103–43.

Newton, M.J. 1999. Precedent autonomy: life-sustaining intervention and the demented patient. *Cambridge Quarterly of Healthcare Ethics* 8(2): 189–99.

Nozick, R. 1974. *Anarchy, State, and Utopia.* New York: Basic Books.

Nussbaum, M.C. 1986. *The Fragility of Goodness: Luck and Ethics in Greek Tragedy and Philosophy.* Cambridge: Cambridge University Press.

O'Brien, M. 1989. *Anatomy of a Nursing Home: A New View of Residential Life.* Owings Mills, MD: National Health Publishing.

Ohta, R.J. and B.M. Ohta. 1988. Special care units for Alzheimer's disease patients: a critical look. *Gerontologist* 28(6): 803–8.

O'Neill, O. 1984. Paternalism and partial autonomy. *Journal of Medical Ethics* 10: 173–8.

O'Neill, O. and W. Ruddick (eds.). 1979. *Having Children: Philosophical and Legal Reflections on Parenthood.* New York: Oxford University Press.

Pankratz, L. and L. Kofoed. 1988. The assessment and treatment of geezers. *Journal of the American Medical Association* 259(8): 1228–9.

Parks, J.A. 1998. A contextualized approach to patient autonomy with the therapeutic relationship. *Journal of Medical Ethics* 19(4): 299–311.

Parsons, T. 1951. *The Social System.* Glencoe, IL: Free Press.

Parsons, T. 1958. Definitions of health and illness in light of American values and social structure. In E.G. Jaco (ed.), *Patients, Physicians, and Illness: Source Book in Behavioral Science and Medicine.* New York: Free Press, 165–87.

Parsons, T. 1975. The sick role and the role of the physician reconsidered. *MMFQ/Health and Society* 53(3): 257–78.

Pegels, C.C. 1981. *Health Care and the Elderly.* Rockville, MD: Aspen.

Pellegrino, E.D. and D.C. Thomasma. 1981. *A Philosophical Basis of Medical Practice.* New York and Oxford: Oxford University Press.

Pellegrino, E.D. and D.C. Thomasma. 1988. *For the Patient's Good: The Restoration of Beneficence in Health Care.* New York and Oxford: Oxford University Press.

Perry, M.J. 1988. *Morality, Politics and Law.* New York and Oxford: Oxford University Press.

Pignatello, C., M. Taylor, and P.A. Young. 1989. *The Exercise of Autonomy by Older Adults in the Home Care Setting.* Princeton, NJ: Princeton University Press.

Plath, D. 1983. 'Ecstasy years' – old age in Japan. In J. Sokolovsky (ed.), *Growing Old in Different Societies: Cross-Cultural Perspectives.* Belmont, CA: Wadsworth, 147–53.

Portnoi, V.A. 1981. The natural history of retirement: mainly good news. *Journal of the American Medical Association* 245(17): 1752–4.

President's Commission for the Study of Ethical Problems in Medicine and Biomedical and Behavioral Research. 1983. *Securing Access to Health Care*, Volume 1: *Report.* Washington, DC: US Government Printing Office.

Priester, R. 1990. Leaving homes: residents on their own recognizance. In R.A. Kane and A.L. Caplan (eds.), *Everyday Ethics: Resolving Dilemmas in Nursing Home Life.* New York: Springer, 155–64.

Proot, I.M., H.F.J.M. Crebolder, H.H. Abu-Saad, and R.H.J. Ter Meulen. 1998. Autonomy in the rehabilitation of stroke patients in nursing homes. A concept analysis. *Scandinavian Journal of Caring Science* 12: 139–45.

Proot, I.M., H.H. Abu-Saad, W.P. de Esch-Janssen, H.F.J.M. Crebolder, and R.H.J. Ter Meulen. 2000a. Patient autonomy during rehabilitation: the experiences of stroke patients in nursing homes. *International Journal of Nursing Studies* 37: 267–76.

Proot, I.M., H.F.J.M. Crebolder, H.H. Abu-Saad, T.H.G.M. Macor, and R.H.J. Ter Meulen. 2000b. Facilitating and constraining factors on autonomy: the views of stroke patients on admission into nursing homes. *Clinical Nursing Research* 9: 460–78.

Proot, I.M., H.F.J.M. Crebolder, H.H. Abu-Saad, T.H.G.M. Macor, and R.H.J. Ter Meulen. 2000c. Stroke patients' needs and experiences regarding autonomy at discharge from nursing home. *Patient Education and Counseling* 41: 275–83.

Quante, M. 1999. Precedent autonomy and personal identity. *Kennedy Institute of Ethics Journal* 9(4): 365–81.

Quante, M. 2000. Personal identity as basis for autonomy. In G.K. Becker (ed.), *The Moral Status of Persons*. Atlanta, GA: Rodopi, 67–75.

Rabin, D.L. and P. Stockton. 1987. *Long-Term Care for the Elderly: A Factbook*. New York and Oxford: Oxford University Press.

Rest, J., D. Cooper, R. Coder, et al. 1974. Judging the important issues in moral dilemmas of development. *Developmental Psychology* 10(4): 491–501.

Rich, B.A. 1996. The values history: restoring narrative identity to long-term care. *Journal of Ethics, Law, & Aging* 2(2): 75–84.

Richards, D.A.J. 1981. Rights and autonomy. *Ethics* 92(1): 3–20.

Rieff, P. 1966. *The Triumph of the Therapeutic: Uses of Faith After Freud*. New York: Harper & Row.

Riesman, D. 1950. *The Lonely Crowd: A Study of the Changing American Character*. New Haven, CT: Yale University Press.

Robb, B. 1968. *Sans Everything: A Case and Answer*. London: Nelson.

Rogers, C. 1974. Dependence and counterdependency in psychoanalysis and religious faith. *Zygon* 9: 190–9.

Rosenfelt, R.H. 1965. The elderly mystique. *Journal of Social Issues* 21(4): 37–43.

Roth, H.L. 1890. *The Aborigines of Tasmania*. London: Kegan, Paul, Trench, Trubner.

Roth, J.R. 1973. Care of the sick: professionalization vs. love. *Science, Medicine and Man* 1: 173–80.

Rothman, D.J. 1971. *The Discovery of the Asylum: Social Order and Disorder in the New Republic*. Boston: Little, Brown.

Sabatino, C.P. 1989. *Final Report: The Impact of Patient/Client Rights Regulations on the Autonomy of In-Home Care Consumers*. Washington, DC: American Bar Association, Commission on Legal Problems of the Elderly.

Sabatino, C.P. 1990a. Client-rights regulations and the autonomy of home-care consumers. *Generations* 14(Supplement): 21–4.

Sabatino, C.P. 1990b. *Final Report: Lessons for Enhancing Consumer-Directed Approaches in Home Care*. Washington, DC: American Bar Association, Commission on Legal Problems of the Elderly.

Sailors, P.R. 2001. Autonomy, benevolence, and Alzheimer's disease. *Cambridge Quarterly of Healthcare Ethics* 10(2): 184–93.

Sandel, M. 1982. *Liberalism and the Limits of Justice*. New York: Cambridge University Press.

Sartre, J.P. 1966. *Being and Nothingness*. H.E. Barnes (tr.). New York: Washington Square Press.

Savishinsky, J.S. 1991. *The Ends of Time: Life and Work in a Nursing Home*. New York: Bergin & Garvey.

Saxton, M. 1981. Are women more moral than men? An interview with psychologist Carol Gilligan. *Ms* 10(6): 63–6.

Scarry, E. 1985. *The Body in Pain: The Making and Unmaking of the World*. New York and Oxford: Oxford University Press.

Scheler, M. 1972. *Ressentiment*. W.W. Holdheim (tr.). New York: Schocken Books.

Schneider, M.D. and L. Oliver. 1987. *North Dakota Long Term Care Facilities Admission Contract Terms: Survey of North Dakota Nursing Homes*. Bismark, ND: Legal Assistance of North Dakota.

Schutz, A. 1967. *The Phenomenology of the Social World*. G. Walsh and F. Lehnert (trs.). Evanston, IL: Northwestern University Press.

Schutz, A. 1970. *Reflections on the Problem of Relevance*. R.M. Zaner (ed.). New Haven, CT: Yale University Press.

Schutz, A. 1971a. *Collected Papers, I: The Problem of Social Reality*. M. Natanson (ed.). The Hague: Martinus Nijhoff.

Schutz, A. 1971b. *Collected Papers, II: Studies in Social Theory*. A. Brodersen (ed.). The Hague: Martinus Nijhoff.

Schweitzer, M. 1983. The elders: cultural dimensions of aging in two American Indian communities. In J. Sokolovsky (ed.), *Growing Old in Different Societies: Cross-Cultural Perspectives*. Belmont, CA: Wadsworth, 168–78.

Searle, J.R. 1983. *Intentionality: An Essay in the Philosophy of the Mind*. Cambridge: Cambridge University Press.

Selye, H. 1956. *The Stress of Life*. New York: McGraw-Hill.

Shanas, E. 1979. Social myth as hypothesis: the case of the family life of old people. *Gerontologist* 19(1): 3–9.

Sher, G. 1987. Other voices, other rooms? Women's psychology and moral theory. In E.F. Kittay and D.T. Meyers (eds.), *Women and Moral Theory*. Totowa, NJ: Rowan & Littlefield, 178–89.

Shield, R.R. 1988. *Uneasy Endings: Daily Life in an American Nursing Home*. Ithaca and London: Cornell University Press.

Siegel, J. and C. Taeuber. 1986. Demographic dimensions of an aging population. In A. Pifern and L. Bronte (eds.), *Our Aging Society: Paradox and Promise*. New York: W.W. Norton, 79–110.

Slater, P. 1970. *The Pursuit of Loneliness.*, Boston, MA: Beacon Press.

Sommer, R. 1969. *Personal Space*. Englewood Cliffs, NJ: Prentice-Hall.

Sommers, C.H. 1987. Filial morality. In E.F. Kittay and D.T. Meyers (eds.), *Women and Moral Theory*. Totowa, NJ: Rowan & Littlefield, 69–84.

Spitz, R. 1965. *The First Year of Life*. New York: International University Press.

Straus, E.W. 1963. *The Primary World of the Senses: A Vindication of Sensory Experience.* New York: Free Press of Glencoe.

Straus, E.W. 1966. *Phenomenological Psychology.* New York: Basic Books.

Subcommittee on Law and the Elderly. 1987. *Maryland Nursing Home Contracts: A Manual for Residents and Advocates.* Baltimore, MD: Maryland State Bar Association.

Tagliaczzo, D.L. and H.O. Mauksch. 1979. The patient's view of the patient's role. In E.G. Jaco (ed.), *Patients, Physicians, and Illness*, Third Edition. New York: MacMillan, 185–201.

Taylor, C. 1976. Responsibility for self. In A.O. Rorty (ed.), *The Identity of Persons.* Berkeley and Los Angeles: University of California Press, 281–99.

Taylor, C. 1979. What's wrong with negative liberty? In A. Ryan (ed.), *The Idea of Freedom: Essays in Honour of Isaiah Berlin.* Oxford: Oxford University Press.

Taylor, E.A. 1981. *Draft Report. Unnamed Nursing Home Investigation.* Seattle, WA: Federal Trade Commission.

Thomasma, D.C. 1984. Competency, dependency, and the care of the very old. *Journal of the American Geriatrics Society* 32: 906–14.

Toulmin, S. 1981. The tyranny of principles. *Hastings Center Report* 11(6): 31–9.

Toulmin, S. 1990. *Cosmopolis: The Hidden Agenda of Modernity.* New York: Free Press.

Townsend, C. 1971. *Old Age: The Last Segregation.* New York: Grossman.

Tulloch, J.C. 1975. *A Home is Not a Home* (*Life Within a Nursing Home*). New York: Seabury.

Twaddle, A.C. 1979. The concept of health status. In E.G. Jaco (ed.), *Patients, Physicians, and Illness*, Third Edition. New York: MacMillan, 145–61.

Uhlenberg, P. 1987. A demographic perspective on aging. In P. Silverman (ed.), *The Elderly as Modern Pioneers.* Bloomington, IN: Indiana University Press.

VanDeVeer, D. 1986. *Paternalistic Intervention: The Moral Bounds of Benevolence.* Princeton, NJ: Princeton University Press.

van den Berg, J.H. 1966. *Psychology of the Sickbed.* Pittsburgh, PA: Duquesne University Press.

Veatch, R.M. 1981. *A Theory of Medical Ethics.* New York: Basic Books.

Veatch, R.M. 1982. Medical authority and professional medical authority: the nature of authority in medicine for decisions by lay persons and professionals. In G.J. Agich (ed.), *Responsibility in Health Care.* Dordrecht, Holland: D. Reidel, 127–37.

Vesperi, M. 1983. The reluctant consumer: nursing home residents in the post-Bergman era. In J. Sokolovsky (ed.), *Growing Old in Different Societies: CrossCultural Perspectives,* Belmont, CA: Wadsworth, 225–37.

Vladeck, B.C. 1980. *Unloving Care: The Nursing Home Tragedy.* New York: Basic Books.

Warshaw, G.A., J.T. Moore, S.W. Friedman, et al. 1982. Functional disability in the hospitalized elderly. *Journal of the American Medical Association* 248(7): 847–50.

Watson, W. and R. Maxwell. 1977. *Human Aging and Dying: A Study in Sociocultural Gerontology.* New York: St Martin's Press.

Wellman, C. 1985. A *Theory of Rights: Persons Under Laws, Institutions, and Morals.* New York: Rowman and Allenheld.

Wetle, T. 1995. Ethical issues and value conflicts facing case managers of frail elderly people living at home. In L.D. McCullough and N.L. Wilson (eds.), *Long-term Care*

Decisions: Ethical and Conceptual Dimensions. Baltimore and London: Johns Hopkins University Press, 63–86.

Whitbeck, C. 1985. Why the attention to paternalism in medical ethics? *Journal of Health Politics, Policy and Law* 10: 181–7.

White, R.W. 1959. Motivation reconsidered: the concept of competence. *Psychological Review* 66: 297–333.

White, R.W. 1960. Competence and the psychosexual stages of development. In M.R. Jones (ed.), *Nebraska Symposium on Motivation.* Lincoln, NB: University of Nebraska Press, 97–141.

Whitehead, A.N. 1948. *Science and the Modern World.* New York: Mentor Book.

Woodward, K. 1986. Reminiscence and the life review: prospects and retrospects. In T.R. Cole and S.A. Gadow (eds.), *What Does It Mean To Grow Old?* Durham, NC: Duke University Press, 137–61.

Yeats, W.B. 1959. *The Collected Poems of W.B. Yeats.* New York: MacMillan Company.

Young, P.A. 1990. Home-care characteristics that shape the exercise of autonomy: a view from the trenches. *Generations* 14(Supplement): 17–20.

Young, P.A. and M. Pelaez. 1990. The In-Service Education Program of the Home Health Assembly of New Jersey. *Generations* 14(Supplement): 37–8.

Young, R.B. 1980a. Autonomy and 'inner self'. *American Philosophical Quarterly* 17(1): 35–43.

Young, R.B. 1980b. Autonomy and socialization. *Mind* 89: 565–76.

Young, R.B. 1986. *Personal Autonomy: Beyond Negative and Positive Liberty.* New York: St Martin's Press.

Zaner, R.M. 1981. *The Context of Self: A Phenomenological Inquiry Using Medicine as a Clue.* Athens, OH: Ohio University Press.

Zerubavel, E. 1979. *Patterns of Time in Hospital Life.* Chicago and London: University of Chicago Press.

Zerubavel, E. 1981. *Hidden Rhythms: Schedules and Calendars in Social Life.* Chicago and London: University of Chicago Press.

Further reading

Adler, J.E. 1987. Moral development and the personal point of view. In E.F. Kittay and D.T. Meyers (eds.), *Woman and Moral Theory.* Totowa, NJ: Rowan & Littlefield, 205–34.

Baier, A. 1985. *Postures of the Mind: Essays on Mind and Morals.* Minneapolis: University of Minnesota Press.

Belson, B.S., J.C. Dopkeen, and W.A. Getchell. 1988. Meeting employees' needs for elder care. *Compensation and Benefits Management* 4(2): 117–21.

Bergsma, J. and D.C. Thomasma. 2000. *Autonomy and Clinical Medicine: Renewing the Health Professional Relation with the Patient.* Dordrecht: Netherlands: Kluwer Academic Publishers.

Binstock, R.H., L.E., O. Cluff, and von Mering (eds.). *The Future of Long-Term Care: Social and Policy Issues.* Baltimore, MD: Johns Hopkins University Press, 1996.

Bishop, C.E. and S.L. Karon. 1989. The composition of home health care expenditure growth. *Home Health Care Services Quarterly* 10(1/2): 139–75.

Booth, T. 1986. Institutional regimes and induced dependency in homes for the aged. *Gerontologist* 26(4): 418–23.

Braun, J.V. and S. Lipson (eds.). *Toward a Restraint-Free Environment: Reducing the Use of Physical and Chemical Restraints in Long-Term and Acute Care Settings.* Baltimore, MD: Health Professions Press, 1993.

Brock, D.W. 1988. Paternalism and autonomy. *Ethics* 98: 550–65.

Buchanan, A.E. 1981. Medical paternalism. In M. Cohen, T. Nagel, and T. Scanlon (eds.), *Medicine and Moral Philosophy.* Princeton, NJ: Princeton University Press, 214–34.

Burrow, J.A. 1988. *The Ages of Man.* Oxford: Oxford University Press.

Butler, R. 1974. Successful aging and the role of the life review. *Journal of The American Geriatrics Society* 22(12): 529–35.

Childress, J.F. 1982. *Who Should Decide? Paternalism in Health Care.* New York and Oxford: Oxford University Press.

Christie, R.J. and C.B. Hoffmaster. 1986. *Ethical Issues in Family Medicine.* New York: Oxford University Press.

Cohen, E.S. 1985. Autonomy and paternalism: two goals in conflict. *Law, Medicine and Health Care* 13(4): 145–50.

Cohler, B.J. 1983. Autonomy and interdependence in the family of adulthood: a psychological perspective. *Gerontologist* 23(1): 33–9.

Cole, T.R. 1987. Class, culture, and coercion: a historical perspective on longterm care. *Generations* 11(4): 9–15.

Cole, T.R. and S. Gadow (eds.). 1986. *What Does It Mean To Grow Old? Reflections From the Humanities.* Durham, NC: Duke University Press.

Donchin, A. 1984. Personal autonomy, lifeplans, and chronic illness. In L. Smith (ed.), *Respect and Care in Medical Ethics.* Lanham, MD: University Press of America, 23–44.

Frankfurt, H. 1976. Identification and externality. In A. Oksenberg Rorty (ed.), *The Identities of Persons.* Berkeley, CA: University of California Press, 239–51.

Garfinkel, H. 1967. *Studies in Ethnomethodology.* Englewood Cliffs, NJ: Prentice-Hall.

Germain, C.B. 1984. The elder and the ecology of death: issues of time and space. In M.T. Tallmer, E.R. Prichard, A.H. Kutscher, R. Debe, M.S. Hale, and I.K. Goldberg (eds.), *The Life-Threatened Elderly.* New York: Columbia University Press, 195–207.

Gubrium, J.F. (ed.). 1976. *Time, Roles and Self in Old Age.* New York: Human Sciences Press.

High, D.M. 1988. All in the family: extended autonomy and expectations in surrogate-health care decision-making. *Gerontologist* 28(Supplement, June): 46–51.

High, D.M. and H.B. Turner. 1987. Surrogate decision-making: the elderly's familial expectations. *Theoretical Medicine* 8: 303–20.

Hill, T.E. Jr. 1987. The importance of autonomy. In E. Feder Kittay and D.T. Meyers (eds.), *Women and Moral Theory.* Totowa, NJ: Rowan & Littlefield, 129–38.

Hurka, T. 1987. Why value autonomy? *Social Theory and Practice* 13(3): 361–82.

Husserl, E. 1962. *Ideas: General Introduction to Pure Phenomenology.* W.R. Boyce Gibson (tr.), New York: Collier Books.

Jecker, N.S. (ed.). 1991. *Aging and Ethics: Philosophical Problems in Gerontology.* Clifton, NJ: Humana Press.

Jonsen, A.R. and S. Toulmin. 1988. *The Abuse of Casuistry: A History of Moral Reasoning.* Berkeley and Los Angeles: University of California Press.

Kalish, R. 1979. The new ageism and the failure models: a polemic. *Gerontologist* 19: 398–402.

Kane, R.L. and R.A. Kane. 1982. *Value Preferences and Long Term Care.* Lexington, MA: E.C. Heath.

Kastenbaum, R. 1968. Perspectives on the development and modification of behavior in the aged: a developmental perspective. *Gerontologist* 8: 280–4.

Kastenbaum, R. 1969. What happens to the man who is inside the aging body? An inquiry into the developmental psychology of later life. In F.C. Jeffers (ed.), *Duke University Council on Aging and Human Development. Proceedings of Seminars,* 1965–1969. Durham, NC: Duke University Press, 99–112.

Kastenbaum, R., V. Durbin, P. Sabatini, and S. Artt. 1972. 'The ages of me': toward personal and interpersonal definitions of functional aging. *International Journal of Aging and Human Development* 3: 197–211.

Katz, J. 1984. *The Silent World of Doctor and Patient.* New York: Free Press.

Katz, P.R., R.L. Kane, Mezey, and D. Mathy (eds.). 1995. *Quality Care in Geriatric Settings: Focus on Ethical Issues.* New York: Springer.

Kohlberg, L. 1973. Continuities in childhood and adult moral development revisited. In P. Baltes and W. Schaie (eds.), *Lifespan Developmental Psychology: Personality and Socialization.* New York: Academic Press, 179–204.

Kohlberg, L. 1981. Moral development, religious thinking and the question of a seventh age. In *Philosophy of Moral Development.* New York: Harper & Row, 311–72.

Komrad, M.S. 1983. In defense of medical paternalism: maximizing patient autonomy. *Journal of Medical Ethics* 9: 38–44.

Kupfer, J.H. 1990. *Autonomy and Social Interaction.* Albany, NY: State University of New York Press.

Lidz, C.W. and R.M. Arnold. 1990. Institutional constraints on autonomy. *Generations* 14(Supplement): 65–8.

Mahowald, M.B. 1980. Against paternalism: a developmental view. *Philosophy Research Archives* 6, No. 1386.

Mahowald, M.B. An alternative to paternalism. Unpublished manuscript.

Mattiasson, A.-C. 1995. *Autonomy in Nursing Home Settings.* Stockholm, Sweden: Karolinska Institute.

Mauss, M. 1967. *The Gift: Forms and Functions of Exchange in Archaic Societies.* New York: Norton.

Merelman, R.M. 1984. *Making Something of Ourselves: On Culture and Politics in the United States.* Berkeley and Los Angeles: University of California Press.

Mezey, M.D., C.K. Cassel, M.M. Bottrell, K. Hyer, J.L. Howe, and T.T. Fulmer. 2002. *Ethical Patient Care: A Casebook for Geriatric Health Care Teams.* Baltimore, MD: Johns Hopkins University Press.

Miller, B.L. 1981. Autonomy and the refusal of lifesaving treatment. *Hasting Center Report* 11(4): 22–8.

Moody, H.R. 1985. Ethics and aging: old answers, new questions. *Generations* 10(2): 5–9.

Moody, H.R. 1987. Ethical dilemmas in nursing home placement. *Generations* 11(4): 16–23.

Neu, J. 1977. *Emotion, Thought and Therapy.* Berkeley and Los Angeles: University of California Press.

Nisbet, R. 1975. *Twilight of Authority.* New York: Oxford University Press.

Norton, D.L. 1976. *Personal Destinies: A Philosophy of Ethical Individualism.* Princeton, NJ: Princeton University Press.

Olson, E., E.R. Chichin, and L.S. Libow (eds.). 1995. *Controversies in Ethics in Long-Term Care.* New York: Springer.

O'Neill, O. 1989. *Constructions of Reason: Explorations of Kant's Practical Philosophy.* Cambridge: Cambridge University Press.

Pincoffs, E.L. 1986. *Quandaries and Virtues: Against Reductionism in Ethics.* Lawrence, KS: University Press of Kansas.

Proot, I.M., H.H. Abu-Saad, L.G.J. Van Oorsouw, and J.J.A.M. Stevens. 2002. Autonomy in stroke rehabilitation: the perceptions of care providers in nursing homes. *Nursing Ethics* 9(1): 36–50.

Rai, G.S. (ed.). 1999. *Medical ethics and the Elderly: A Practical Guide.* Amsterdam, Netherlands: Harwood Academic Publishers.

Rappaport, M. and J.B. Wood. 1989. Financing and home health agencies. *Home Health Care Services Quarterly* 10(3/4): 131–47.

Rorty, A.O. (ed.). 1976. *The Identities of Persons.* Berkeley, CA: University of California Press.

Rothman, D.J. 1980. *Conscience and Convenience: The Asylum and Its Alternatives in Progressive America.* Boston: Little, Brown.

Rowles, G.D. and R.J. Ohta (eds.). 1983. *Aging and Milieu: Environmental Perspectives on Growing Old.* New York: Academic Press.

Ruddick, S. 1989. *Maternal Thinking: Toward a Politics of Peace.* Boston: Beacon Press.

Scheler, M. 1973. *The Nature of Sympathy.* P. Heath (tr.). Hamden, CT: The Shoe String Press.

Schneewind, J.B. 1997. *The Invention of Autonomy: The History of Modern Moral Philosophy.* Cambridge: Cambridge University Press.

Schutz, A. 1971. *Collected Papers, III: Studies in Phenomenological Philosophy.* I. Schutz (ed.). The Hague: Martinus Nijhoff.

Schutz, A. and T. Luckman. 1973. *The Structures of the Life-World.* R.M. Zaner and H.T. Engelhardt Jr (trs.). Evanston, IL: Northwestern University Press.

Scott, G.E. 1990. *Moral Personhood: An Essay in the Philosophy of Moral Psychology.* Albany, NY: State University of New York Press.

Sennett, R. 1980. *Authority.* New York: Alfred Knopf.

Shanas, E. 1968a. The family and social class. In E. Shanas, P. Townsend, D. Wedderburn, H. Fris, P. Milhoj, and J. Stchouwer (eds), *Old People in Three Industrial Societies.* New York: Atherton Press, 227–57.

Shanas, E. 1968b. The family as a social support system in old age. *Gerontologist* 19: 169–74.

Shanas, E. and G.F. Streib (eds.). 1965. *Social Structure and Family: Generational Relationships.* Englewood Cliffs, NJ: Prentice-Hall.

Sheehy, G. 1977. *Passages: Predictable Crises of Adult Life.* New York: Bantam Books.

Sherman, E. and E.S. Newman. 1981. The meaning of cherished personal possessions for the elderly. In R. Kastenbaum (ed.), *Old Age On the New Scene.* New York: Springer, 240–51.

Shils, E. 1981. *Tradition.* Chicago, IL: University of Chicago Press.

Simon, Y. 1980. *A General Theory of Authority.* Notre Dame, IN: University of Notre Dame Press.

Singer, P. 1979. *Practical Ethics.* Cambridge: Cambridge University Press.

Singer, P. (ed.). 1986. *Applied Ethics.* Oxford: Oxford University Press.

Spicker, S.F. 1978. Gerontogenic meditation: memory, dementia and medicine in the penultimate years. In S.F. Spicker, K.M. Woodward, and D.D. Van Tassel (eds.), *Aging and the Elderly: Humanistic Perspectives in Gerontology.* Atlantic Highlands, NJ: Humanities Press, 153–80.

Spicker, S.F. and S.R. Ingman (eds.). 1984. *Vitalizing Long-Term Care: The Teaching Nursing Home and Other Perspectives.* New York: Springer.

Straus, E.W., M. Natanson, and H. Ey. 1969. *Psychiatry and Philosophy.* M. Natanson (ed.). New York: Springer-Verlag.

Thomasma, D.C. 1983. Beyond medical paternalism and patient autonomy: a model of physician conscience for the physician–patient relationship. *Annals of Internal Medicine* 98: 243–8.

Tinetti, M.E., D. Baker, W.T. Gallo, A. Nanda, P. Charpentier, and J. O'Leary. 2002. Evaluation of restorative care vs usual care for older adults receiving an acute episode of home care. *Journal of the American Medical Association* 287: 2098–105.

Tocqueville, A. de. 1969. *Democracy in America.* G.W. Lawrence (tr.). New York: Doubleday, Anchor Books.

Toulmin, S. 1982. How medicine saved the life of ethics. *Perspectives in Biology and Medicine* 25(4): 736–49.

Trattner, W.I. and W.A. Aschenbaum (eds.). 1983. *Social Welfare in America: An Annotated Bibliography.* Westport, CT: Greenwood Press.

Van Tassel, D. and P.N. Stearns (eds.). 1986. *Old Age in a Bureaucratic Society.* Westport, CT: Greenwood Press.

Weiner, M.B. 1984. Aging as ongoing adaptation to partial loss. In M.T. Tallmer, E.R. Prichard, A.H. Kutscher, R. Debe, M.S. Hale, and I.K. Goldberg (eds.), *The Life-Threatened Elderly.* New York: Columbia University Press, 31–9.

Wertheimer, A. 1987. *Coercion.* Princeton, NJ: Princeton University Press.

Williams, B. 1973. A critique of utilitarianism. In J.J.C. Smart and B.Williams (eds.), *Utilitarianism: For and Against.* Cambridge: Cambridge University Press, 75–155.

Williams, B. 1976. Of persons, character, and morality. In A.O. Rorty (ed.), *The Identity of Persons.* Berkeley and Los Angeles: University of California Press, 197–216.

Williams, B. 1985. *Ethics and the Limits of Philosophy.* Cambridge, MA: Harvard University Press.

Index